EARLY BIRDS
FLOCK TOGETHER

Joys, Sorrows–and Laughs–in Senior Living

For Barb –
a fellow
United Methodist
woman!
Nancy Renner

Orange Hat Publishing
www.orangehatpublishing.com - Waukesha, WI

EARLY BIRDS
FLOCK TOGETHER

Joys, Sorrows–and Laughs–in Senior Living

Nancy Runner

Orange Hat Publishing
www.orangehatpublishing.com - Waukesha, WI

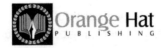

Dedicated to my children, Alex and Abby.

Table of Contents

Chapter 1
Snow Angel

The empty bird feeder nagged at my conscience. A black-capped chickadee bobbed toward the empty tray and then darted away. "I'm coming, I'm coming," I mumbled as I pulled on my son Alan's 30-year-old silver moon boots that he wore in fifth grade. A calm December day, in the thirties—I felt comfortable in my jeans and blue corduroy big shirt—and I didn't even need a jacket. The glare of sunlight on the snow made me think of my sunglasses, but I didn't turn back to get them. In one hand, I held an old metal Christmas pail decorated with holly and candy canes. It once contained potato chips, but now it stored sunflower seeds. I liked it because it had a handle. My other hand held the peanut butter suet.

I tiptoed through the knee-deep snow to the feeder in my front yard, stepping as if on a freshly-mopped kitchen floor. The feeder was placed to see birds through the picture window, but that meant trekking about ten feet from the front sidewalk. Finally at the feeder, I poured sunflower kernels through the wooden hatch into its glass-front and then began to undo the twist-tie that locked the suet cage from prying squirrels. Twisting the wire, I leaned back slightly on my heels. Once the rubber-coated cage opened, I needed to remove the suet out of its plastic. The cellophane wouldn't cooperate, and I tilted further and further back. As I tried to tear it with my cold hands, my center of gravity failed me, and there was nothing to grab onto to stop my fall. Surprised, I found myself on my back in the snow like a beetle. When I tried to push myself up, my hands plunged through the unresisting snow like beaters through soft peaks of whipped cream.

Gloves would have been a good idea.

I craned my neck to search my front yard and neighborhood.

No one in sight.

Usually, my street was busy. My next door neighbor, Julie, might call 'hello' or wave as she shoveled her walk; Steven worked in his front yard, landscaped to look like an English garden; Kathy and Tom exercised their yellow lab while they pushed their baby in the stroller or hopped into their car to run errands.

I bought my three-bedroom Cape Cod fifteen years ago, after my divorce. Having my own space made me feel like a competent, independent woman. But now I needed help.

There was not a soul to be seen. It was a weekday, and I remembered most of the neighborhood activity took place on weekends when people were home from work. Oh, where was kind Dawn when I needed her? This past fall, she surprised me by coming across the street while I was raking. She brought her rake with her.

"You've got a lot of leaves, Nancy," she had said.

Then she began piling them into the street with long sweeping motions. I couldn't believe how fast younger people rake. It would have taken me hours without her help.

Now here I was, stuck in the snow. I heard my daughter, Amanda's, worried voice in my head.

"Mom, you should always take your cell phone when you go out!"

The sky gazed down on my plight with genial, pale-blue eyes. "Sorry." It seemed to say. "You're on your own."

To get out of this predicament, I would have to help myself.

You can do it, Nancy, I thought. *Remember, you are a competent, independent woman.*

Finally, I managed to turn on my side and then all fours, but I still couldn't muster the strength to stand. Instead, breathing hard, I crawled through the snow like an infantrywoman toward my front sidewalk.

You <u>had</u> to put the bird feeder in the middle of the yard so you could see the birds better through the window.

At last, my clammy red hands found the cement steps, and one shaky knee bent enough to give me a foundation. From there, I grasped the next step and, finally, stood upright. The used-to-be-blue jeans and shirt were entirely white. I looked like a powdered-sugar donut.

My eyes returned to the snowy yard, and I saw an inelegant tunnel; the formerly smooth expanse of snow was now marred by my flailing snow angel.

Forget the suet. But that metal pail will rust.

I took a couple of careful steps to retrieve the seed bucket, shaking the snow off. My breathing slowed.

Note to self: move the feeder closer to the sidewalk.

Once back inside, I sat at the kitchen table with my head in my hands and ignored the puddles growing around my boots. It took a few more moments before I could brush the snow off, run my hands under warm water, and make a cup of tea. I would need to mop the floor.

It's been twenty years since Arthur and I parted ways. But today was the first time I really felt alone.

***

My fall in the snow set wheels in motion. Perhaps I knew I was going to put my house on the market. Perhaps it was even in the back of my mind when I started renovations this past year. I wanted to get a few things done before I retired from my job at an insurance company. I loved living here. It has been *my own house.*

My renovations were nothing fancy. They were just meant to blend with my solidly middle-class neighborhood in the city of Milwaukee. My neighbors consisted of firefighters, police officers, and teachers. But the Cape Cod house built in the '50s needed freshening. New kitchen floor, sink, and countertops. The fixture over the kitchen table was dated, and the imitation yellow brick linoleum floor looked scratched. The kitchen looked much better after installing new white/gray linoleum "tiles." Over the years, I had re-sided the house and put in a brick walkway from the front porch to the backyard. I'll miss that. It made my yard look more like an English garden. And I will miss my new composite granite kitchen sink. Hopefully, any future buyer will love it as much as I have.

I couldn't afford a complete makeover, but a new medicine cabinet and light fixture really spruced up my one bathroom. A few years ago, I had the tub reglazed, and now it looked like new.

I was in a good position to list the house after the Christmas holidays. The timing was right. The real estate market was starting to recover. Marge, who lived down the street, has had her house on the market for the past six months, but it still has the yellow linoleum floor from the 1950s and wall-to-wall brown shag carpet. I hoped my updates would make a difference. Nowadays, buyers want a home that is move-in ready.

I didn't intend to buy another house. Condos were a possibility, but those had to be kept updated to keep them desirable for future buyers. Please, no more remodeling. Condos also have unpredictable association fees, and special assessments can wreak havoc on a budget if major repairs crop up—such as a new roof or plumbing problems.

Apartment living seemed to be the most attractive option. Not that I have lived in an apartment since I was newly-married, but it might be appropriate now. I made appointments to tour a couple of 55+ complexes, as well as those with no age restrictions. I wasn't sure if I wanted to live around all ages (loud parties and music?), but I would give them a look.

I did the math. Here, I paid a man to snow plow the driveway, but the steps and sidewalk were my responsibility. All of the payments added up: cleaning the gutters, trimming trees, and, of course, mowing lawns and putting mulch down once spring arrived. If the furnace died, it was on me. Did I mention property taxes? Even though the mortgage would soon be paid off, there were still a lot of expenses. Paying rent wouldn't be too much different. I would just have fewer responsibilities and even fewer worries.

Amanda asked me to look at some 55+ complexes in Westown, where she lived, so I agreed to do that, too. That would mean moving away from Milwaukee and starting over—new church, new doctors, new friends. Of course I visited my daughter in Westown many times but had not thought of living there. It would be great to be close to her family, and they had no other relatives close by. My grandchildren in Westown, Nate and Anna, were eleven and seven at the time—nice ages since they still wanted to spend time with Grandma. Compared to Milwaukee with its population of 500,000, Westown's 70,000 seemed more manageable. Also, there was a local two-year university in Westown, which offered interesting programs and classes.

In Milwaukee, I had Alan, Jane, and my grandsons Blake, who was eight, and Joseph, who was four, just three miles away. But Jane had her mother, sister, and brother in town, with lots of cousins for the boys to play with.

Amanda's kids didn't have any family nearby. It would

still be an easy drive from Westown back to
to visit Alan, Jane, and my longtime friends there.

As I discovered when I fell in the snow, the neighbors
worked and often weren't around. It wasn't like the old
days when I raised kids in a Milwaukee suburb and there
were lots of children in the neighborhood, along with
stay-at-home moms. Now, I was definitely on my own.

I've been in the same bridge group for twenty-five years.
We used to look forward to retirement and imagined all the
free time we would have to get together for lunch. Now
we could hardly get a foursome together. The gals were
always off somewhere visiting grandchildren or traveling.

The monthly book group I'd been in for thirty years
completely fell apart. It started with the "Newcomers
Club" when many of us moved to Milwaukee thirty
years ago. Two of the stalwart members died and several
moved to warmer climes. But there were book groups
everywhere, so I didn't doubt I could find a new one
wherever I moved.

I grew up moving often since travel was part of my
dad's job, and I always enjoyed exploring a new town
and meeting new people. I lived in Illinois and Maryland

growing up, but I also lived in England and Argentina. I met Arthur in college in Iowa. The two of us lived in Iowa, Oklahoma, Minnesota, and Ohio before moving to Wisconsin. Still, I didn't want to minimize the upheaval I would experience by moving out of town at this phase in my life. After all, I lived in Milwaukee for thirty years, and change doesn't come easily for "senior" citizens.

Isn't moving one of the top ten stressors? Oh, wibble, wobble, wibble, wobble, there are so many things to think about.

Ariane de Bonvoisin, the author of *The First 30 Days*, says people who navigate change successfully have these traits:

1. They have a positive outlook. They're confident they can change and optimistic that life is on their side.

2. They believe that, whatever the change, something good will come from it.

3. They believe they are resilient and strong and can get through anything.

4. They acknowledge change will stir feelings of fear, doubt, impatience, blame, shame, and guilt, but they don't let that stop them.

5. They let go of the idea of how life "should" be and cultivate acceptance. When they feel stuck, they focus on empowering thoughts and look for the opportunities change creates.

6. They know they are connected to something bigger than themselves.

7. They look within to find their calm, unchanging center.

8. They seek support from helpful, knowledgeable people who can reduce their sense of isolation.

9. They take action. They have a plan, they move forward, and they take care of their health during this stressful period.[1]

***

I was busy! The house would go on the market in five days. I listed with Debbie Noels, an active agent in the area. She was very complimentary about all of my updates to the house and said, "It only takes one." By that, she

---

[1] Used with the author's permission. For more information about Ariane de Bonvoisin please go to her website http://www.arianedebonvoisin.com/

meant it only takes one right buyer. Fingers crossed.

I had a nice Christmas with Amanda and her family, and we visited Bentwood Hills, which is the 55+ apartment complex only one mile from their house. It had great curb appeal—a brick three-story building with white balconies and seasonal landscaping of miniature fir trees and red balls. Many of the residents had decorations or lights on their balconies which gave a festive air to the entire complex. But I hoped to be in a more walkable area with access to the grocery store, coffee shops, etc. In most big cities, you can walk to a market and buy your food for the day. That appealed to me, but I didn't think I'd have that option in the suburbs.

I planned to return to Westown later that month. Amanda had two more places to show me.

In Milwaukee, I visited *Briarwood* Hills, which was owned by the same company as *Bentwood* Hills. Briarwood was in a suburb about twelve miles west of where I lived, so it was quite a drive to play bridge or visit Alan and his family. It was attractive, though, and they offered scads of activities for their residents, from book clubs to bridge.

I decided against "all ages" apartment communities. I visited two and realized I was looking for the activities offered at 55+ properties. In a regular apartment, I would still be alone, and many of the other residents would be gone all day at jobs and school. At "senior" apartments, you can participate or not, but at least there were opportunities to gather with your neighbors. After my experience floundering in the snow, I wanted to be around people.

I visited the Lutheran Home, which was close by, and that was way too old for me. You're required to eat one meal a day in their dining room. I was not ready for that. I also visited Eastown which had a wonderful location in downtown Milwaukee and transportation to plays and concerts. But they required over one hundred thousand dollars upfront as something called an "endowment" and, again, the monthly rent included unnecessary services, like housekeeping and linen changes. My idea of independent living was doing my own cooking and vacuuming. And I'd take care of my own bed, thank you very much.

Chapter 2
The Big Move

When I told Amanda about my decision to move to Westown, she said, "Really?!" I could hear the happiness in her voice. My decision felt right to me, too. What a relief.

To seal the deal, I drove there again, and we toured two properties she had in mind. One was near a mall, which was good for shopping and walking, but had the most obnoxious man as property manager; while we were there, a resident came into his office to change dollars for quarters to do laundry, and the manager commented, "Ha, ha. You can see I'm the boss. No one can do their laundry without me!"

Plus, I would rather not pay to do laundry in coin-operated machines. I guess I'm a little fastidious, but you never know what guy just had his tighty-whities in there! The units also had window air conditioners. If I could afford it, I'd prefer central air. We couldn't get out of there fast enough.

The second property we visited was gorgeous, with an ice cream parlor and pool table for the residents, but their idea of independent living, again, was my idea of assisted living. I was not ready for a meal program or transportation services. Those amenities raised the rent to over three thousand dollars per month. I might keep it in mind for ten years down the road if I need to file a claim on my long-term care policy.

The housing journey finally ended at Bentwood Hills. I loved the idea of being just one mile from Amanda and her family, even if it meant driving to do my shopping. Every decision has its drawbacks. My mother moved from Oklahoma to Milwaukee to be near us when she was seventy—my age now. She lived only thirty minutes away, and that seemed close at the time, but it turned out to be difficult when she started showing signs of dementia and I drove back and forth frequently—sometimes twice a day.

At Bentwood Hills, their monthly newsletter was filled with activities. They had a monthly dinner/social-type event, as well as bridge groups, knitting groups, book clubs, chorus and, of course, Bingo. The day I play Bingo is the day you can shoot me. It sounded so old! My sister in California, who was only sixty-three and loved Bingo, said I was a Bingo snob. She's probably right.

The fireside room at Bentwood was lovely, with a big gas fireplace surrounded by comfy chairs and a sofa. There was a kitchen where residents could prepare potluck suppers, birthday celebrations, etc. The community room could handle sixty to seventy people for special dinners. Since this was independent living, there was no meal program. Good. No paying for unnecessary services.

I loved the library. It was filled with bookcases, hundreds of books, computer and printer, a red leather chair with matching ottoman, as well as a couch and a coffee table stocked with daily newspapers and the Wall Street Journal.

There was even a small theater with black leather chairs and a big-screen TV for movies. And a popcorn machine, of course. My grandchildren would love that. There was an exercise room equipped with a treadmill, stationary bike, and weights. I didn't know how often I would use that, but it was there. And a beauty parlor— very convenient when it was snowing outside.

Heated underground parking! That would be needed in central Wisconsin. It was funny that I was moving north when most people my age were moving south. Bentwood had central air and no endowment required, just monthly rent. It was simply senior apartments for those who were 55+. It was not part of a continuum of care with assisted living and nursing home all on one campus. If the day comes when I need assisted living, I will have to move.

When Mother moved into independent living at her retirement home, many of the residents at her place were older and teased her good naturedly about being such a youngster. Then, they told her they wished they had made the move sooner. Her philosophy was always, "Do what you have to do before you have to do it."

I've been told the average age at Bentwood is mid-seventies.

It was going to be a new adventure, that was for sure. I was putting a positive spin on this big change—selling my own home I bought after our divorce and moving away from the city I had lived in for more than thirty years. Part of aging gracefully, to me, was realizing that accepting change becomes more difficult with each passing year. It won't get easier as I age.

I don't want to be one who says, "I should have done this sooner."

***

I drove back to Westown and looked at available apartments at Bentwood Hills. A two-bedroom, two-bath would be available April 1st, so I took it. I hoped that wasn't an April Fools' Day omen.

And my house sold! The closing was on the fifth of March, and the buyer agreed to let me rent from her for the rest of the month. The buyer was a young woman who taught in the Milwaukee Public Schools. Selling the house was a bit harrowing, especially dealing with her inspector.

He left a device in the basement for twenty-four hours to test for radon gas. I never thought of radon gas, so I did not know what to expect. It was a relief when he got a very low reading, one of the lowest he had ever seen. But then he informed me that my garage was in danger of collapsing—something about lacking proper support beams. I almost fell over. Did that mean I needed a new garage? My handyman, Todd, came over and looked. "Yep," he said. "Whoever installed the original garage door opener cut one of the main beams."

"Well, for heaven's sake," I said. I'd lived there fifteen years and never noticed a problem. I was about to burst into tears. But then Todd told me he could jack up the roof and install a new beam. Bless him. That cost me less than three hundred dollars. Unexpected news of that nature is so stressful. Now, everything seemed to be coming together.

I knew what I would be doing until moving day—packing! And making trips to Goodwill. Somehow, I had to get rid of all of the stuff in the basement and garage, plus the third bedroom.

It was a good thing I downsized once already when I sold the house Arthur and I owned. And I never used the attic at my place. Still, there was so much stuff—boxes of Alan and Amanda's treasures and school papers, boxes of books I never opened when I moved to this house fifteen years ago, boxes of Christmas decorations; the list goes on and on.

***

I finally moved to Bentwood Hills, and it was such a relief.

I *never* worked so hard in my life and, believe me, if I ever move again they will take me out feet first. Bless my friend Connie, who made eight trips to Goodwill with her car loaded to the gills. Alan helped by getting all of his remaining boxes out of the basement. And he took the mower and snow blower, as well as other gardening implements I would no longer need. Amanda came to town to clean the stove and empty the refrigerator.

Still, how on earth do we accumulate so much *stuff*? As I unpacked I thought—*why did I want this*? And *which box is that in*? It was going to be a process to get settled, but at least the furniture was all in place and I could start to relax. I really liked my apartment and the cozy living room with gas fireplace. It was so nice to have a washer and dryer just steps away, all on one level. The walk-in shower was a treat, too, and felt very safe. The huge bedroom closet was a ridiculous luxury. Of course, it was designed to accommodate a couple, and I was just one person, so it was more than enough hanging space. My luggage and card table set were stored in there, too.

It was an adjustment not having a kitchen island. That's where I used to eat breakfast. In my new apartment, I ate breakfast and lunch at the dining room table and dinner on a tray while I watched the news.

Living in a place with other people was a comfort. At night, the light from the hallway could be seen under my entryway door. For some reason, I found this reassuring.

My neighbors asked me where I was from and if I had family nearby. They assured me that I'd soon be able to find the office, library, or game room without getting lost.

When people introduced themselves, they'd say, "Don't worry if you don't remember my name. We all have to introduce ourselves several times before it sticks."

I could relate to that. Some people didn't even bother with names. They'd say, "Hi, neighbor." Or, "Good morning, friend."

My underground parking spot was very convenient—it was nice to get into a car that wasn't too cold or too hot.

One day I drove into the garage and met a light blue sedan coming toward me. The driver was going about five miles per hour because he had a large white plastic bag of garbage balanced on his hood—directly in front of him! I could see his shock of white hair and watery, pale eyes through the windshield, peering around the bag.

"What the...?"

Soon, I realized his motivation. I, too, have taken a bag of garbage in my car and planned to drop it off in the trash area on my way out of the garage. More than once I forgot to drop off the garbage and drove around running my errands with the bag still in the car. Once, I had it next to me on the passenger seat and took it to church with me.

We seniors are a creative bunch when it comes to dealing with short-term memory issues.

Chapter 3
Expiration Dates

My friend's son posted a picture on Facebook of all the bottles of cocktail sauce he had removed from her refrigerator.

Yes, there were a few bottles, but probably not more than six or seven. And yes, some of them were past their "expiration dates," but it was cocktail sauce! We all know how acidic tomatoes are.

This may have struck a nerve with me since Amanda cleaned out my cupboards and refrigerator before the move.

I contended that the "sell by" date does not mean the "use by" date, but she was the "Kitchen Police" and made me throw away perfectly good food.

It seems the Food and Drug Administration requires expiration dates on everything—not only dairy products and meat, but things like envelopes of onion soup mix and bottles of vinegar. Those items last forever.

After the way Amanda purged my cupboards, I couldn't

find a can of tomato soup when I needed it for a recipe. Luckily, my next door neighbor had a can—reduced-sodium, which I prefered. Too bad I didn't look at the expiration date until after I ate my dinner. It expired *six* years ago. I was still alive, though, which proved my point.

Speaking of expiration dates, I like this poem reminding us some attitudes need to perish as well.

Expiration Dates[2]
by Debra Monthei Manske of South Milwaukee

Don't use the mayo after that day.
Toss the eggs on this one.
Little numbers say a new beginning is due.
Little dates say, "All done, move on."
Too bad grudges don't come stamped with a date
or meanness suddenly find itself expired.
Nastiness needs a time to be tossed,
bad feelings find a day to be healed.
Like on that old bottle of mayo,
shadowy dates could suddenly appear in the air
little numbers to tell us when
enough's enough.

2 Used with the author's permission. Contact dmontheimanske@hotmail.com.

***

Our staff planned a Mother's Day event for the residents, and I felt excited to attend my first activity. For ten dollars per person, we were invited to dress in our finest and enjoy catered appetizers, small sandwiches, a chocolate fountain with fruit, and a choice of beverages. My granddaughter Anna, Amanda, and I attended, and we delighted in the harp music, which provided lovely background without overwhelming the conversation. Anna said she wanted to be a harpist when she grew up.

White tablecloths covered the round tables in the community room. Place cards reserved our seats.

The staff stayed late to throw this extravaganza, and they dressed in formal attire. Our marketing director wore a little black dress and black hat with a veil. The property manager looked splendid in a long, flowing black gown, and she went from table to table offering wine refills for our glass stemware.

The three of us enjoyed the chocolate fountain, pinwheels, veggies and dip, as well as a selection of ham and Swiss or turkey and American cheese sandwiches on buns.

The property manager also took pictures of each family group as a memento.

I was feeling quite happy with my decision to move here, until, at the table next to us, a woman complained she didn't like the wine. Leaving her glass of wine untouched except for a sip, she went to the bar and asked for a complimentary Bloody Mary. Back at her table, she ate the olives on her swizzle stick and took a big gulp. Then she declared, "This vodka is cheap!"

She left that drink, too, and went back to the bar to ask for something else. All of this was loud enough to be noticed at nearby tables.

As we left, we overheard a group of ladies in the hallway grumbling about the sandwiches. Something about them not being what they expected.

Hello? For ten dollars you could scarcely buy one glass of wine at a restaurant. Caterers and harpists have to eat, too. The sandwiches were delicious, and I have the seven-year-old granddaughter to prove it. She ate two.

It must be discouraging for the staff to plan a unique

event and then hear grumbling. As I looked for new friends, I hoped I could find some who had an "attitude of gratitude." I hoped I hadn't moved to Grumpy Town!

***

I took baby steps getting acquainted in my new town. I wanted to find a church home as soon as possible.

After visiting several churches in the area, I observed something I never noticed before—most people sat at the ends of the pews. Perhaps they wanted to be the first ones out of the door, or they were preparing for a bathroom emergency, but very few slid over to the middle of the pew. This meant the pew was "blocked" for anyone else to sit there unless you crawled over the end-sitters.

I admit to claiming the end of the pew at weddings for a good view of the bride as she walks down the aisle. But the rest of the time I tried to scoot to the middle so other worshippers could join me.

One church held a potluck luncheon after the service. When I went to the social hall, many chairs were tilted on the tables to indicate those places were saved. I felt unwelcome. It seemed strange to see adults still save seats like sixth-graders. Why are people so resistant to sitting with someone new?

I was sure I would find the right church soon. But it wasn't easy to meet new people when you were seventy years old. I remember how much fun my neighbor Connie and I had when our children played together, and we drank coffee and kept our eyes on them. Children are great at breaking the ice for adults. I maintain that all mothers of young children are lonely and need other women friends with whom they can have an adult conversation. And as we get older we continue to need social opportunities. That was why I was glad I moved there—it was nice to see people as I walked around the building. I just needed to find the right ones!

Chapter 4
Living Outside the Box

There were 150 apartments at Bentwood Hills. Thirty-eight of them were occupied by couples, and there were eight single men. That meant 104 apartments were occupied by single women—widows, divorcees, and a few who never married. Just think—each of these women had a story to tell. I once wrote my story in the following essay:

"Living Outside the Box"

"I see you checked the 'married' box, as well as the 'single' box, and the 'divorced' box," my new doctor observed.

"That's correct," I said. "I've been all three."

She peered at me over her glasses.

At the doctor's office, at the bank, on insurance forms, everyone wants to know your marital status. If I check the 'single' box, it's true. I have been single again, since my divorce twenty years ago. When a doctor sees the "married" box checked, does she know if the couple is happy or miserable? And if there is a status box titled "divorced," what does the reader conclude? Is the divorced person a loser, a victim, a promiscuous hussy, or a survivor?

Anyone who decides to end a thirty-year marriage might be called courageous, or perhaps foolhardy. It isn't easy to start over after investing thirty years in a relationship.

How did I arrive at the epiphany that led me to divorce?

Have you ever poured out your heart to your Higher Power?

It was on my fiftieth birthday, with my thirtieth wedding anniversary only a few weeks away. A lot of people do some soul-searching on their fiftieth birthday, and I was no different.

My husband was out of town on business, and my two teenage children were out of the house. I sat in my quiet living room and this is what I said, out loud:

"I want You to know I am expecting to earn a gold star," I told God. "After thirty years of this, through thick and thin, I sure hope there is at least a special medal."

Arthur and I weren't happy—had not been for many years. I thought about divorce at year twenty and year twenty-five, but who doesn't go through bad patches? I had been seeing marriage counselors for at least ten years, and sometimes my husband went along. However, in his mind, I was the one who needed professional fixing.

Like many women of my generation, I lost myself somewhere along the way in my marriage. It began early. Arthur and I met as college students. We dated a few times, and I remember one of those early afternoons when we were in his car.

"Let's go meet my parents!" he said. (He was a commuter student.) I protested.

"I'm not dressed! I don't want to meet them like this." (I was in my cut-off jeans and red college sweatshirt.)

"It'll be fine. They won't mind."

I was mortified. *I* minded. This was not the way to make a good first impression. I protested a few more times, but my misgivings were shrugged away. In short order, we were at his home and I, red-faced at my appearance, tried to "fake it" with a big smile.

Sure enough, Arthur told me later, his dad asked that

evening if he was in a hurry to marry me because I was pregnant. With that big red sweatshirt, I could have been hiding something. I felt mortified again. I was an old-fashioned girl who believed sex came after marriage. But they didn't know that.

This should have served as a warning to me. In our marriage, my wishes and feelings were often pooh-poohed as inconsequential.

Another early sign: I would have liked to have kept my maiden name along with my new married name. Not hyphenated—it was the '60s after all. Just use my maiden name as a middle name. My new father-in-law-to-be asked my intentions. He was very contemptuous of women who held onto their maiden names. I wanted to please him, so I said, "No, I will now be Nancy Elizabeth Runner." He nodded his approval.

We were still college students when we married. I remember I felt sad at my college graduation, which my father attended, to see all connection to him and his name eliminated when my diploma was announced. He was the one who continued to pay for my college education even after I married.

After my father's death, I was in my thirties and changed my Social Security card and all my public record information to show my maiden name as a middle name. I wanted my birth name to continue, not just be dropped forever. I still cared what my father-in-law thought, but I had matured enough to recognize his beliefs originated from insecurities about strong women. No one gave me any grief about the change I made, and probably would not have at the time of our marriage if I had had more gumption.

I did not stand up for myself when I was twenty years old. I am sure other women can identify with me when I say it was very important to my husband that I always agreed with him—in public especially, but also at home.

My opinions were inferior or unreasonable. If I complained about Arthur's stacks of business papers on our bedroom dresser, he responded, "There are many widows who would love to have their husband's mess around again."

How wrong of me to be so petty.

I know many women must be subservient to their husbands and are not "permitted" to be educated or seek employment. I was fortunate to have an education. My husband did not want me to work while we had young children at home, and I was happy to be at home with them during their early years. Once they were in school, I wanted more. Our pastor counseled us and said to Arthur, "It is difficult for many women who have been successful in school to be satisfied with just homemaking and child rearing. If Nancy had a full-time job, there would be changes at home. You might eat out more and perhaps pay for a housekeeper. How does that sound to you?"

I was ready to say, "Sign me up!" But Arthur frowned and shook his head.

Many years later, as I sat in the chair in my living room, the babies were teenagers, and our marriage was worse. I returned to work, finally, in a local medical office and enjoyed contributing to the family income. However, Arthur was so "out of love" with me, he could hardly stand to be in the room with me, and he suffered from stomach problems and migraines.

I thought I was doing the brave and selfless thing, sticking it out and trying to change myself and my attitudes, recognizing I was the only one I could change.

That is how I came to ask God for a gold star like my first-grade teacher used to paste on the top of my spelling test. After all, we probably had twenty or thirty more years of this marriage ahead of us.

Then something happened I was not expecting. I felt a still, small voice say to me, "But I wanted you to enjoy your life."

Wait a minute. This stopped me in the middle of my thought. I wasn't one to hear voices; however, these words, "But I wanted you to enjoy your life," had definitely not come from me.

You will notice that the voice did not say, "But I wanted you to get a divorce," only that I was supposed to enjoy my life. I had choices in this matter. Somehow, I needed to find a way to enjoy my life as it was or find the courage to make a drastic change. In a very human way, I made a decision that in order to enjoy my life, our sham of a marriage needed to end.

The next day, I asked Arthur to move out. He expressed surprise but agreed. It was easier than I thought. He actually began looking for apartments that weekend, causing my therapist to comment, "That's the fastest he ever did anything you wanted." He was as unhappy as I was. When I faltered in my resolve and said, "Maybe we are making a mistake," he told me, "No, I can see myself starting a new life."

I know I was fortunate. Many women do not own property. I was the joint owner of our home. With my education, I believed in myself and believed I could find a job. In the United States, I had opportunities that would not be available to women in other countries. Although I was afraid of the unknown future, I had enough faith in myself and God to believe things could be better. I did not want to "settle" any longer.

We divorced after the required waiting period, without attorneys. Our city had an organization that helped couples to divorce "pro se," (Latin for "by oneself") for one hundred and fifty dollars. Can you imagine this in other parts of the world? Many women are stuck in arranged marriages and have no right to initiate divorce. We had no significant assets to wrangle about and wanted to make the separation as amicable as possible. Arthur agreed to pay child support for three years until Amanda turned eighteen. Our house did not have much equity in it, and Arthur signed it over to me. I took over various credit card debts to make up the difference.

And here I have to say how lucky I was, again, to live in a country with a fairly modern medical system. Not that it is the best in the world by any means, but I was fortunate to have planned the size of my family. To me, birth control is the secret to lifting women out of poverty. We had two children, and our family was a manageable size to allow me to think about myself and re-entry into the corporate world. So many women are in a cycle of constant pregnancies which can ruin their health and tie them to the home because childcare expenses make working out of the question.

There is no good time for divorce when it comes to the children. My husband and I were typical of those couples who stay together "for the kids." I can't say if it was right or wrong. Our children were blindsided by our separation since we never quarreled in front of them. Afterward, they talked together as brother and sister do, and said, "Of course. We should have recognized that they avoided each other. Dad never came to the dinner table!"

of our friends were shocked, too. We were active members of our church. It just proved my point that checking the "married" box on an application tells nothing about the mental health of the couple in that marriage. Most unhappy couples don't talk about their grievances—too much shame and embarrassment about not making their relationship work.

One of my husband's coworkers suggested we hold a "Ceremony of Forgiveness." This was something new to me, but she explained that the divorcing couple could say words of forgiveness to each other, either in front of a clergy person at church or in the privacy of their own home. I agreed to follow the ceremony my husband brought home, provided we could do it informally, sitting around our dining room table. There was an actual bulletin, an order of worship, like you might see in a church, with our names at the top of the page. It began with these words:

The purpose of this ceremony is to heal hearts, by forgiving the past and releasing the future. This rite is to be held in the presence of the couple's children.

Nineteen-year-old Alan sat with us while we did this,

but fifteen-year-old Amanda would have nothing to do with it. We didn't insist she participate.

The "Ceremony of Forgiveness" went on to say:

We join in God's presence, as we hereby let go the bond of marriage between us. We ask God's blessing, as we both seek and grant forgiveness. We join in the recognition that through the grace of God there are no endings but only the chance for new beginnings, and we pray this day for God to give that new beginning, to us and to our children.

There was a time for each of us to speak to each other and say words of thanks. Alan also spoke and told us he felt grateful for the family in which he grew up.

Words of prayer followed, including these:

May the golden cord that has bound the two of us in marriage be not violently severed, but lovingly, carefully, and peacefully laid aside, this act forgiven by God . . . never shall the bond of marriage be made meaningless, before God or humankind . . . May these two beloved children of God remember that the love of this union was important, and honor it always.

We ended with Arthur saying these words to me:

Nancy, I bless you and release you. Please forgive me. I forgive you. Go in peace. You remain in my heart through the grace of God.

I said the same words to him. As we stood from the dining room table, Arthur grasped my hand and said, "It is important for me to know you forgive me."

Once again, I said, "I forgive you." Yes, I had the thought, "What, exactly, am I forgiving you for?" But I didn't ask because it didn't matter.

Alan was distracted by his new college life. He later married a young woman whose parents were also divorced, and that seemed to help them forge a connection. Amanda was angry for a few years, but her dad made concerted efforts to stay in touch, taking her out to dinner and staying interested in her life. She lived with me for a while after she left school, before getting an apartment with a coworker. The time we shared helped us grow closer. I have to be honest and say I was ready for "the kids" to adjust to the new reality after many years of considering them first. I know my attitude was "deal with it."

No matter how well divorce is handled, there are

profound losses when a marriage ends, as well as surprising "finds."

First, I lost my extended family. No more brother-in-law, Robert. No more niece, Jessica, or nephew, Paul. Thirty years of history—poof! Up in smoke. I bit my tongue instead of chiming in, "Oh, my husband's family was from Wyoming, too." I no longer said, "My mother-in-law quilts."

Of course, the word "husband," spoken with a certain pride of partnership, was lost. And, I lost some of our shocked "couple" friends. Divorce might be contagious.

When I read the obituaries, I often saw these words: *She was the beloved wife of*—I felt sad I was no one's beloved.

My engagement diamond and gold wedding band were as good as lost—baubles couldn't sparkle from inside a dark drawer where they rested in their cotton-lined coffin.

Half our furniture left—the oak dresser that was his grandmother's, the cherry tilt-top table he liked, the watercolor "Loons over the Lake" that used to hang over the sofa, and the maple bedroom set from our guest room.

Going to a party or restaurant, I missed being dropped off at the door while Arthur parked the car. It was harder to make my own entrance, but I learned to put on a smile and walk into the room.

Arthur had a good head for directions, so I counted on him to read maps. He used to plan our vacations. I learned to look over the brochures to see what appealed to me. But now, thank goodness GPS came along.

There were things I didn't miss, like his cereal bowl in the sink with dried-on Raisin Bran and sour milk in the bottom. He could never be bothered to rinse the bowl.

Before our divorce, I breathed air polluted with unspoken anger and recrimination. We were strangers in the same house—seldom speaking, never touching.

After the judge's final decree, I lost the tight feeling in my chest, the ever-present anxiety that poisoned me— surely an ulcer or colon cancer in the making. I found the freedom to make my own decisions and have my own opinions.

No, I am not saying it was easy. Making a fresh start meant selling our suburban home and moving to a smaller one by myself in the city. It meant going from a family-friendly, laid-back employer to looking for a job with more career opportunities—at fifty years old.

I started a new job with benefits, earned promotions, and retired at age sixty-six with my own pension. I absolutely loved working. And here I would like to say something about women in the workforce. They are needed. They bring communication skills and inclusiveness to the job. I remember when women first started to tear down barriers, and some men said, "No man will want to work for a woman."

Now, in the younger generation, it comes naturally. Some women are good bosses and some aren't, just like men.

It would be a travesty if women went back to having no choices. Some women may choose full-time homemaking, and that is their prerogative. For others, and I am one of them, working outside the home is stimulating. In a perfect world, women and men could work, stay at home with small children as needed, and re-enter the workforce without penalty. Greater flexibility would benefit both men and women. Some politicians want to go back to the days of women having no access to birth control and being at home full-time. This would be a loss for businesses as well as for families. It is important for women to fight for the right to safe and effective birth control, quality childcare, and family-sensitive work environments.

As for me, instead of being punished for my failed marriage, as some religions warn, I thrived. Perhaps it was a by-product of our "Ceremony of Forgiveness," but Arthur and I were able to go our own ways without much disdain. Today, twenty years later, I am reluctant to say anything negative about our marriage. After all, our children and grandchildren are products of it. A minister who provided us marriage counseling said, "God is continuing to bless you in your new life."

There are still things that are hard. Weddings are difficult. It's painful to see hopeful, young couples vowing to stay together "until death do us part." It is a reminder of failure. After all, we met as starry-eyed college students and thought we could face anything as long as we were together. I loved the way he solved problems spontaneously, never worrying about the future. He thought I was spunky and industrious. I've heard "opposites attract, and then repel." That was true in our case.

Recently, our couple-friends have begun to celebrate their fiftieth anniversaries. Our fiftieth would have been last year. They endured. We didn't. A few of them appear to have admirable marriages, but many don't. I feel a twinge of failure on our anniversary, but I quickly get over it.

Some wonder if I am lonely. An unhappy marriage can feel desolate when there is a person in the other room but you don't know how to connect with them. That is loneliness. After our divorce, I tried online dating once, but let my membership lapse after the trial period. There were too many men like the one whose profile said, "Lunch without sex is like a man in the desert without water."

I remember the day I came home from working at my new job and took off my coat in my 1950s, 1,000-square-foot Cape Cod home. I walked into my cozy living room, decorated in white wicker with French blue and yellow slipcovers. It was cheerful—and my own space. I recognized a feeling of peace that engulfed me.

Yes, I was alone, but not lonely. Sometimes I imagined myself speaking to a group of women, telling them I live in 1,000 square feet of my own home, which I own, with no man telling me what to do. I can picture how they cannot even believe such a thing is possible. Truly, I know I am fortunate compared to most women around the world.

Arthur joined a singles group and met a woman who became his wife a couple of years later. I was glad he married someone our age and didn't go for a new wife twenty years younger. We sometimes share grandparent duties, and our exchanges are cordial.

There have been positive changes, in surprising ways. As a teenager, I kept journals but did not write during the thirty years of our marriage. Putting unhappiness down on paper seemed to make it permanent, and I always hoped there would be more "ups" to cancel out the "downs."

After our separation, I resumed journal writing, which helped me work through the challenges of being alone again. My new career called for professional writing in letters, newsletters, and project work. After retiring, I attended writing workshops and joined a supportive weekly writers' group. I have written over one hundred essays, self-published three nonfiction books, and had a few poems and essays published. Grandchildren, singing, and volunteering enrich my life. I recently went kayaking for the first time.

Twenty years have passed since I had that conversation with God in my living room and that moment of epiphany. God wanted me to enjoy my life and I hope God is pleased. Although there have been losses, I have found peace, happiness, freedom, and independence.

Recently I found this poem by Raymond Carver. It helps me feel I, too, am beloved.

Late Fragment

And did you get what
you wanted from this life, even so?
I did.
And what did you want?
To call myself beloved, to feel myself
beloved on the earth.

That's why I struggled in my doctor's office when faced with choosing the 'married,' 'divorced,' or 'single' status box. I have been each one, and each has contributed to who I am today. No status box can capture the fullness of my life. I wish all women could enjoy the same opportunities and freedom.

Chapter 5
Mistaken Identity

I needed Kleenex. At the grocery store, I picked up some chewy high-fiber bread and a bottle of Merlot that was on sale. Then I headed for the perimeter where the meat, dairy, and produce were stocked.

A frowning woman peered into other people's carts.

"Someone took my cart," I overheard her say.

I got out of her way, continued shopping, checked out, and went home.

As I unpacked my groceries, I noticed something odd. *How did Wonder Bread get in here? Wait. What's this? I never buy Hot and Spicy Cheetos.*

Yes, I bought bread, but this loaf was the soft, squishy type of "wheat"—white bread colored with raisin juice. Ugh. There was a bottle of wine, but not Merlot. I grabbed the receipt. $15.99 for white zinfandel? Was that even possible? And Cheetos? I recognized the rest of the groceries, but how odd to have these rogue intruders!

The realization quickly dawned on me. *I was the culprit*

who switched carts with the annoyed lady in the store! But, here was the really scary thing . . . I *checked out* and didn't even notice what I placed on the conveyor belt!

She could still be there looking for her cart. Next week, I'll go to a different grocery store. And you know, I forgot the Kleenex.

***

A new couple moved in—Evangeline and Rupert. Evangeline knocked on my door looking for someone. She couldn't remember the name of the person or apartment number she wanted.

"The lady with the windmill," she said.

With that clue, I thought of Julia, who has a windmill on her patio, so I walked Evangeline to that apartment. Julia greeted us and told me the two were cousins.

"Evangeline has memory problems," she whispered.

I remember how confusing it all was when I first moved in, so hopefully, Evangeline will adapt in time.

Mildred and Trudy have been welcoming to me. Mildred is tall and wears slacks and sweaters. Trudy is short, round, and favors sweatpants. They do everything together.

Mildred knew of a church that served a three dollar chicken dinner once a month. They invited me to go along with them, and we drove around a while before we found the church in a neighboring town. Mildred drove and Trudy rode shotgun. When Mildred had to make a left turn at an uncontrolled intersection, she asked Trudy to look to the right and tell her when it was clear.

"You're good to go now," Trudy said.

"Well, I am not good this way," Mildred replied.

"How is it now? I'm clear to the left."

"No," said Trudy.

"'No' means no cars are coming?" asked Mildred, still watching to the left.

"No, 'no' means don't go—there's a truck coming," warned Trudy.

I closed my eyes in the backseat.

After a while, we saw the church. We figured we were at the right place because there were a lot of cars there. I anticipated the meal ahead.

There would be the usual folding chairs at long tables

and the meal would probably be chicken pieces cooked in mushroom soup, mashed potatoes, salad, and assorted desserts. I really looked forward to the dessert selection. Maybe some lemon bars?

Just as we found a parking place, Mildred saw a distinguished looking man in a dark suit. She rolled her window down and asked him, "Is this the monthly chicken dinner?"

He responded, "No, that's next week. The ladies of the church are providing a reception for Harriet Stewart's funeral."

We turned around and got out of there before you could say "Jack Spratt." On the way home, Trudy said, "Well, we saved three dollars. Want to come over for frozen pizza?"

***

My son-in-law Justin said I moved to central Wisconsin at the ideal time. The summer weather was gorgeous, sunny, and in the seventies. They only get a few ninety-degree days here.

I started some herbs from seeds purchased at Ace Hardware—an economy pack of five different herbs in one box—basil, oregano, parsley, dill, and rosemary. The seeds sprouted in the light through my patio door, plus two strategically placed small lamps.

They survived transplanting into two pots. Since basil is particular and doesn't tolerate any temps lower than fifty degrees, I put that pot out during the day and brought it in at night. Yes, I fussed and babied, and they rewarded me by flourishing.

My patio is a great addition to the apartment's living space. It is large enough for two chairs, an umbrella table, and lots of plants. I miss the bird feeders I had at home, but they drop seed and attract rodents, so they are not allowed here. And, of course, there's no danger of elderly residents falling over in the snow by their feeders, like someone we know did! We can have hummingbird feeders, and I do enjoy that; I have seen one ruby-throated type several times.

Now that I am settled, I think about how I'm going to best use my time here. At the "resort," as we refer to Bentwood, I am now in a book club and a bridge foursome. We play bridge in the library, which is such a beautiful extension of our living area. It's nice not to have to "tidy up" like I used to before hosting bridge in my house.

I have met so many new people, and once a month I go out to breakfast with seven other ladies.

In addition, all of the paperwork is complete for me to become a volunteer at the local hospital. They needed references, medical history, TB tests, and so on. I will be working in the volunteer office doing administrative work. Luckily, I used the computer extensively when I worked, so that experience serves me well.

I returned from five days at a writing workshop in Gresham Lake, Wisconsin. One of the other attendees invited me to a writers' group that meet every week right there in Westown. It was exciting to make new connections.

At the conference, I requested double accommodations. (Yes, I was too cheap to pay the additional hundred bucks for a single.) What could go wrong in less than a week of sleeping in the same room with a stranger?

Shortly after I unpacked (saving three drawers in the

six-drawer chest for my roommate), Gladys arrived. She was a tiny woman from Iowa, probably in her seventies or early eighties. I introduced myself with a smile, and said, "Hi, I am Nancy."

Gladys immediately fluttered her hands and twittered, "Oooh, I have a Nancy!"

I watched in bewilderment as she hurried to open her purse, and she pulled out a stuffed animal—an orangutan named "Nancy." Sort of a Beanie Baby orangutan.

She held Nancy up to her face and kissed her quickly three or four times on her orange nose. With care, every single day, she leaned over and arranged Nancy on the pillow of her bed before going to class. During the day, when we knew the cleaning crew would come, Nancy sat on the bedside table, legs crossed.

In bed at night, Gladys hugged Nancy.

Once I got over my initial surprise, I accepted Nancy, the orangutan in the room. And I learned something. I will no longer ask my grandchildren, "Are you planning to take Foxie or Blankie to college with you?" Apparently, it can be done.

***

"I would like to celebrate my birthday by going to a restaurant for lunch, so I'm organizing a group—no gifts, of course! I hope you don't mind buying your own meal. Can you join me?"

That's how I found two carloads of women to go out for my birthday lunch.

The women I invited to my birthday celebration were delighted to go. At Bentwood Hills, there was a community of available friends. I asked ladies from my book club, bridge foursome, and breakfast group.

Yes, Amanda and her family took me out for dinner. And Alan and Jane drove up with the boys to help me celebrate. It was the first time I was able to give them a tour of my new living space, and they were very happy to see me so well-situated. But I like to get together with friends and celebrate, too. So I made it happen.

I learned to "make it happen" years ago when the kids were toddlers and my feelings were hurt by an overlooked Mother's Day. Rather than cry about it, I decided to be clear about what I wanted and expected.

That meant giving Arthur a large paper grocery sack and the recipe for "Chicken in the Chips." He and the kids had fun crushing the potato chips and then shaking the pieces in the sack before baking them. Of course, I bought the potato chips and chicken pieces, but "voilá." I wanted to be served dinner, and I made it happen.

I also reminded my children, "Don't forget your precious mother's birthday is coming up, and handmade cards will be appreciated."

One Mother's Day, I saw some lovely corsages in the grocery store and bought myself one. A gentleman complimented me on it at church, and said, "Whoops, I better get one of those." I just smiled.

My motto is: If there is something that will make you happy, don't expect anyone to read your mind. Why feel sad when I can make it happen?

Joanna, one of my new Bentwood friends called: "It's my birthday, and I want to go out with some friends like you did. Want to come?"

"Absolutely," I said.

Chapter 6
Memories for Sale

It is aggravating to be a competent and able senior citizen, and then have "something stupid" happen that makes you feel totally incompetent.

I made the simple decision to get a car wash at the local gas station. It's not the first time I have gone through this type of car wash. It's especially fun when the grandchildren go along; they like to sit in the enclosed car, squealing, while the suds and rinse cycles go on around them.

This was my first time at this particular car wash.

The problem began at the outside kiosk where you enter your code. I selected the "Ultimate" car wash because I wanted the undercarriage flush.

That proves I knew what I was doing.

The voice inside the box gave me instructions, but they were so garbled and distorted that they were incomprehensible. Never mind. The door rose, and I entered.

I expertly drove between the two tracks because everyone knows the tracks are for the equipment to go back and forth. The lighted sign in front of me advised, "Drive Forward."

There was a barrier. This was no big deal because often in car washes you have to give a little gas and get your wheels properly aligned. So I gave a little gas and proceeded to go up, up, up, about six inches and then came down with a "clunk."

"Clunk" is not what you want to hear in a car wash.

I opened the door and got out to see what was going on. Luckily, the spray had not started. Where was my underbody flush?

My driver's side wheel had gone over a steel block of some sort, and it did not look good.

Somehow, I was now in the car wash at an unfamiliar angle.

The frantic sign blinked, "Back Up!"

Thank goodness no one was in line behind me. I hated to admit it, but I was stumped.

Near the car wash entrance, a balding, uniformed employee was taking a cigarette break. I walked out to him in what I hoped was a dignified manner and stated the obvious: "I need help."

He glanced at me and I saw myself in his eyes—a panicky gray-haired woman who had done god-knows-what in the car wash. From me, his eyes darted to the interior of the car wash, and he saw my car was "somewhat" sideways.

"Oh, boy," he said, stamping out his cigarette. "I sure hope your axle isn't hung up on that."

At my helper's direction, I got back in the car, lowered my window, and he took charge of the car while I sat there. First, through the window, he turned the wheels to the left as far as they would go. I controlled the pedals as he directed me to back up; then he continued turning the wheels, and I reversed. Meanwhile, the annoying sign blinked, "Drive Forward" followed by, "Back Up!" At last, the car was restored to the proper position.

The car wash whirred into action and a few suds landed in my lap as my good samaritan yelled for me to close the windows.

Thankfully, no permanent damage was done, and I received the "Ultimate" car wash. "Ultimate" has another meaning, too. It means "last." And it was the *last* time I was going to that particular wash.

***

I was in my bedroom and thought I heard the door. Evangeline and I ran into each other in the living room, and we both jumped. She was looking for her cousin again, but still can never remember her name or apartment number. She just says, "Where's the lady—" and then she looks around without finishing her sentence. I told her where Julia lives, but she looked at me with a blank stare, so I walked her to the correct apartment.

And locked my door when I returned to mine.

We have 150 apartments here, and I don't know of any resident as confused as Evangeline. I do think her husband should keep a better eye on her.

By the way, if you ask someone, "Do you know Julia?" and they don't, then the description is something like, "You know, she's the one with the white hair and glasses." That results in a lot of blank looks since that describes ninety percent of the residents.

***

My granddaughter Anna, who is eight, gave me a necklace for my birthday. It has a delicate silver chain and a red cardinal pendant. She knows I enjoy birds. I wanted to wear it the next time I saw her, but I could not get the clasp fastened. I need eyes in the back of my head to do it. So the necklace sits on my dresser.

Luckily, I received those catalogs that have all kinds of items you didn't know you needed until you saw it. I ordered "magnetic jewelry clasps" that fasten onto the ends of your necklace, and then all you have to do is put the magnet ends together. Voilá! I couldn't wait to show her I was wearing it.

If future archaeologists discover one of those catalogs, they will find a treasure trove of information about senior citizens in the twenty-first century. For example, senior citizens had balance problems—see the ads for "power grip grab bars" to make the bathroom safe. And to cope with their arthritic sore knuckles, seniors needed specially padded grippers to help them carry bags. (Never mind they didn't have the strength to carry three bags at one time as shown in the picture.)

Those old people had trouble with their vision—you could tell by the assortment of magnifying items advertised. There's a lighted magnifier, a handheld 5X magnifier, a hanging magnifier to wear around your neck for close work, and a full-page magnifier so you could read more than one sentence at a time. I have one of those, but it doesn't work very well. It's hard to keep it at the right distance from the page. The catalog doesn't even mention my favorite magnifier—the 10X mirror for examining your face for new growth!

The archaeologist would conclude older people in this era had trouble opening things. The catalog contained a special ergonomic puller to lift the rings on soup or soda cans. Another three-in-one apparatus handled screw tops, ring pulls, and bottle caps you had to flip open. There was an opener that rotated itself so your hands were out of the way. Yet, somehow, lids seem more difficult today than ever. "Press down and turn" caps are the worst. Followed closely by "squeeze and turn." And don't get me started on "tear here."

I had so much difficulty opening my bottles of vitamins

and painkillers—I left most of the tops loose. Someday I might pour them all into a bowl, like Skittles, and fish out what I need.

Speaking of pills, catalogs offered a wide variety of daily pill organizers. And we older folks needed them! You could get the Sunday through Saturday version, or the twice daily version with slots for morning and afternoon tablets. If those pill boxes were too bulky for traveling, there were water resistant plastic bags, about two inches square, and they were perfect for carrying your daily dosage. I'd been managing my prescriptions in a box marked Sunday–Saturday for some time. Otherwise, I took my pills so automatically I then wonder, *Did I or Didn't I?*

Finally, the archaeologist would note seniors in the twenty-first century had foot problems. And he or she would be right! The catalogs offered diabetic socks, ankle supports, long-handled toenail scissors for those with trouble bending over, ergonomic clippers for those whose hands tend to slip, special toe separators for those whose toes have been cramped in pointy shoes for way too many years, and special rubs for sore feet, with lavender or Epsom. Those feet were more than seventy years old, so no wonder they hurt.

Catalog companies found a veritable bonanza in the special needs of senior citizens. I loved my magnetic necklace clasps, and I was considering a long-handled appliance to apply lotion to my back. "Comes with six replaceable pads!" It was a long, itchy winter.

***

There is a parallel universe we mortals tend to ignore—and I am not talking about the spiritual world. Long after the human species self-destructs on earth, the residents of this parallel world will continue to thrive.

Yes, I am talking about insects.

Even as I wrote this, a fruit fly darted into the lighted area of my computer screen, then frisked away despite my clumsy efforts to grab it in my fist or smack it against the keyboard. The fruit fly is a marvel of creative engineering. How can such a small body contain a complete nervous and circulatory system? But along with the complex anatomy of this seemingly indestructible master evader came my misery as one fruit fly after another aimed for my ears or nose.

The "melacoryphus lateralis," or seed bug, periodically drives residents of California crazy. Those small red and black insects are so plentiful that residents sweep away piles of their dead bodies or use a leaf blower.

In Wisconsin, there is a similar phenomenon along the Mississippi River when the mayflies hatch. The swarm last summer looked like a rainstorm on radar. The insects diminished visibility and made the roads so slick they caused car accidents.

I attended "The Lakefly Writers' Conference" in Oshkosh, Wisconsin. They branded themselves based on the annual spring infestation around Lake Winnebago. Now that is making lemonade out of lemons—actually using those pesky lake flies as a positive distinction. Hey, you may have the University of Iowa Writers' Workshop, but we have the lake fly—well, I just don't know if that works as a title that's supposed to draw people in.

Hornets loved my patio umbrella. Every morning I approached the umbrella with one timid finger and thumb reaching to look inside. Two or three hornets, still a bit too chilled to be threatening, rested in the fabric folds. Sorry to say, I blasted them off with Raid and only then felt secure enough to have my morning coffee outside. Think of the villains in scary apocalyptic movies, like *The Fly*, *Bigfoot*, *King Kong*, or *Godzilla*. BIG is not nearly as scary as tiny and determined. Diseases like malaria or the Zika virus come from the mosquito. The fat bumblebee, nose-deep in my potted petunias, makes me dodge, dart, and slosh my coffee to stay out of his way.

Back to the problem I faced: fruit flies. A Google search suggested vinegar traps. Another said to swat them with an aluminum pie tin. The larger surface ensured a greater success rate than a fly swatter. But nothing worked, and I feared the tiny fruit fly had taken over the lease on my apartment.

Then I concocted a recipe that really did the trick. In a shallow glass pie plate, or similar, place one cup water, a few drops of essential oil (I used "lemon eucalyptus"), and a few drops of Dawn dish detergent. Stir gently to mix. Place this concoction near a light overnight. (I set it on my stovetop and turned on the overhead "night light.") In the morning, I counted thirteen trapped fruit flies and penned a Haiku to celebrate:

Fruit flies trapped in brine
Tiny little asterisks
That flew off the page

The light attracted them to the sweet smelling mixture, and the soapy detergent drowned them. I repeated for several evenings and was finally bug-free!

***

On our community bulletin board, a resident offered two patio chairs for sale. They were lovely chairs, but our patios could only accommodate seating for a couple of people once you added plants and a table. You know they probably moved from a home with a large deck and needed all of the appropriate furniture for entertaining.

That was one of the difficult things about leaving our homes—so many lovely things we could no longer use or have room to store.

Residents clung to their mahogany curio cabinets that didn't fit into the apartment dining rooms, six-foot-long couches that overwhelmed our living rooms, and electric grills. Electric grills sounded like a good plan, but many older folks didn't want to fool with grilling just one hamburger or just one chicken breast. It sounded efficient to grill four pieces of chicken and save some for later, but we didn't do that either. Either we didn't feel like eating grilled chicken four nights in a row, or it seemed too much of a bother.

How sad when one lady advertised her Christmas collection of angels: angel placemats, angel table runners, angel centerpieces. All for only thirty dollars. You know those brought her joy when she decorated for her family. I wish I could tell young mothers, who are often so fretful decorating and baking, that those years won't last forever. There will come a time when Christmas is so quiet there doesn't seem to be a reason to set up a tree. And boxes of Christmas decorations will remain unopened.

Think about the Christmas china—if one is lucky enough to own a set. It's too much trouble to get it out for one person. One of my friends has four children, and, over the years, she purchased four sets of china to "pass on" to them. You can guess what happened. None of the kids want or use china. They like "everyday" dishes or pottery. So my friend will be taking her sets of china to a resale shop where she will get pennies on her investment.

Another resident posted a note on the bulletin board asking if anyone would like her collection of recipes. For free. Just think, forty or fifty years of wonderful recipes collected over a lifetime of raising a family. Certainly, tastes have changed. "Applesauce Salad" was big in the '60s. The ingredients included lemon Jello, applesauce, and cinnamon red hots. You don't see that on the buffet table very often these days.

Recipe files reveal more than what people ate forty years ago. They tell stories about the family. In my loose-leaf notebook of recipes, I had notes saying, "Alan ate this quiche on his first birthday," and "Amanda loved this *Inside Out Ravioli*." I had recipes my mother passed on to me when I was a young bride. She typed them with personal comments. For example, in the instructions for how to roast a turkey, she wrote, "Don't forget to take the package of giblets out of the turkey carcass. Cover the neck and giblets with water and simmer to make a broth for the stuffing. Throw away anything that looks too repulsive to use."

The "For Sale" section on the bulletin board reminded us that part of our lives was over. And it seemed to have gone so fast. I was reminded of something Andy Rooney, from the television show *60 Minutes*, said. "Life is like a roll of toilet paper. The closer you get to the end, the faster it goes."

Chapter 7
Good Sports

Anna played in a T-ball game.

It was a surprise to see the learning that took place, even at this beginning level. The volunteer coaches pitched three or four balls to the kids to give them a feel for hitting a pitched ball. If they were unable to hit, the tee was brought out and they hit off that. *Any* contact with the ball resulted in a base hit, even if it just fell off the tee to the ground.

All fielders were instructed to throw to first base whenever a ball came to them. One eager father called to his son from the sidelines, "Throw it to second!" But the coach walked over and said, "He's fine. Everyone needs to throw to first at this level." Dad replied, "Oh, yeah. Okay. Okay."

There were no outs at this stage in T-ball. Every batter advanced to first and then around the bases on subsequent hits. The last child in the batting order got the thrill of running all four bases.

These are the life lessons I observed:

Line up in your batting order. (That's how to be orderly and take turns.)

Wear a batting helmet. (Don't take unnecessary risks.)

Drop your bat and run to first base. (No need to carry excess baggage when you are trying to get somewhere.)

Step on the bases as you go around, and don't skip home plate. (Do things in the proper sequence.)

Take your batting helmet over to the other team when it's their turn at bat. (Be generous and show good sportsmanship.)

Pick up or catch a hit ball and only throw it to the first baseman. (Learn the basics first and then progress to more advanced skills.)

Crouch in an alert position when you are in the field and pay attention to the batter. (Be ready for opportunities that may come your way.)

Huddle up with your coach at the end of the game. (It's always good to assess and improve.)

If you're the snack person, distribute snacks to the others before you help yourself. (This is how we share.)

The older generation doesn't need to despair. (As

long as there are so many wonderful volunteers, there is hope for the future.)

***

Mildred and Trudy were at coffee hour where they talked about their recent trip to the grocery store. Their conversation was so delightful I went back to my apartment and wrote a story inspired by them. This piece of fiction appeared in the 2017 issue of *Creative Wisconsin Literary Journal*, published by the Wisconsin Writers' Association.

"Friendship by the Slice"

Friends, like married couples, can be as incompatible as oil and water. Mildred and Trudy lived in the same senior apartment building. They had little in common, yet they did everything together. The other residents called them "the odd couple." They were both in that seventy-ninety "difficult-to-tell-your-exact-age" phase of life. Trudy was the short, round one with a ready smile, who never complained about her poor eyesight. Taller Mildred wore a rusty-colored perm and a tight-lipped smile. Trudy liked comfortable sweats, while Mildred preferred slacks with sweaters. She called herself "no-nonsense," but could sound bitter, as when she complained, "I moved here to be close to my kids, but I never see them." On the other hand, Trudy loved planning parties or taking coffee and a homemade treat to the ladies in the retirement-community beauty shop.

Mildred often took Trudy grocery shopping since Trudy had to give up driving. She laughed, "The police are funny about people going over that yellow line." On one weekly shopping trip, Trudy saw that cherry pies were on sale.

"I think I'll get two," she said.

"What do you need two for?" Mildred huffed.

"I can freeze one," said Trudy. "You never know when you might need a nice cherry pie. And these look good."

The two ladies waited their turn at the checkout. Trudy's cart was quite full, with a whole chicken, a chuck roast, fresh asparagus, a bag of oranges, five pounds of potatoes, half a gallon of milk, an angel food cake, a bag of Hershey's chocolate bars (with almonds), and, of course, two cherry pies. Mildred's five frozen TV dinners didn't take up much room in her cart, next to a bag of apples, a six-pack of beer, and a two-liter bottle of cola.

When the checker rang her total, Trudy pulled out her ancient coin purse. She counted the bills and coins but found she was a couple of dollars short.

Mildred plopped her purse on the conveyor belt and pawed in it until she found her wallet. She handed Trudy the dollars she needed.

Around 6:00 p.m., after her spaghetti carbonara frozen dinner, Mildred sat down on her pink, corduroy loveseat with the newspaper. The only other place to sit was a wooden rocking chair that had belonged to her mother. Too much furniture made Mildred nervous. She scanned the paper but soon laid it on the polished mahogany coffee table and looked for something on TV. There was nothing good. Her eye went back to the newspaper on the table. It looked untidy. She took it to the recycling bag in her closet.

She picked up her knitting, but quit after two rows,

rolled the needles and yarn together, and stowed them away in the knitting bag which she put out of sight on the floor by the loveseat. She decided to wander over to Trudy's apartment but first visited the bathroom. A few dots of toothpaste spray on the bathroom mirror caught her eye. Windex and paper towels, stored under the sink for emergencies like this, rubbed the spots off. Then she walked down the hall to Trudy's apartment, just a few doors away.

Trudy was cutting herself a piece of cherry pie, and she offered one to Mildred. As usual, Trudy's dining room table was completely set for six. Today, she displayed a cream-colored tablecloth, matching cloth napkins, white china plates with an ivy pattern around the rim, and sterling silver flatware.

"Why should I have these beautiful things and not use them?" Trudy always said. "Besides, I want anyone who calls on me to know there is a place at the table for them."

A large glass bowl of purple lilacs occupied the center of the table and their fragrance filled the air. Mildred avoided looking into the kitchen, which was a disaster, with cookware and dishes piled in the double stainless steel sink, as well as on the countertops. Just the thought of diminished counter space gave her the heebie-jeebies.

Trudy said, "Let's sit outside and enjoy this beautiful evening."

Her apartment balcony held several chairs and an assortment of clay pots. She enjoyed her herb garden of oregano, basil, and rosemary. Pink petunias and red impatiens nodded on the specially-built white wooden shelves. Mildred thought so many flowers were a waste of money. One pot of geraniums suited her just fine.

"They last longer, look great, and you hardly have to water them," Mildred said.

The two friends enjoyed the mild evening and the sugary-almond taste of the pie mixed with the tart cherries. Trudy bustled around with her coffee pot.

"Can't you just sit still?" Mildred complained.

"Well, you can't have pie without coffee," Trudy laughed.

They reminisced about their grandmothers' cooking methods. Both agreed their grandmothers didn't really use cookbooks but rather followed the old-time measurements of a "pinch" of this or a "handful" of that.

Mildred smiled as she remembered, "Grandmother used to say, 'Add butter the size of an egg.'"

Trudy perked up. "That's interesting. I never heard of anyone buttering the sides of an egg. Why would she do that?"

Mildred put her coffee cup down and looked at Trudy in disbelief. "I didn't say 'butter the sides of an egg.' That's ridiculous. You didn't hear me correctly. Are you wearing your hearing aid? I said, 'Grandma would add 'butter the SIZE of an egg!'"

"Oh!" chuckled Trudy. "That makes more sense."

After about an hour, Mildred stood to go back to her apartment.

"Don't forget those two dollars you owe me," she said.

"Well, you ate a piece of the cherry pie," Trudy blinked behind her thick glasses.

"That was out of the first pie, not the second one I lent you the money for. Besides, it was a small piece."

"I'll pay you next time I go to the bank."

Mildred knew that could be a while.

"Just give me a piece of that pie to take home, and we'll call it even."

Trudy cut Mildred a good-sized slice and lifted it onto a pretty china plate with a platinum rim. She covered it with a red cotton napkin and handed it to her friend, someone who would drive you to the grocery store and lend you money in a tight spot. Mildred accepted the pie. She thought about the extra places at Trudy's dining room table, and the second cherry pie in her freezer.

"See you tomorrow," they both said.

***

Certain experiences just scream "Wisconsin," such as:
- Friday night fish fries
- Dinner at a supper club
- Summer weekends "up north" at a cabin or cottage
- Exploring a lake by canoe or kayak
- Fishing and hunting
- Abundant bird life—observing eagles, hawks, and cranes
- The Brewers and the Packers
- The Wisconsin State Fair

Although I moved here thirty-five years ago, if I want

to be a true Wisconsinite, I still have to check off certain experiences on my Badger State bucket list.

The ubiquitous fish fry requirement was crossed off long ago and on a regular basis. I do love some fried perch with rye bread and cole slaw. Walleye is good, too. Some restaurants offer potato pancakes, but I prefer the twice-baked potato. In this part of the world, Friday is fish night.

Supper clubs are uniquely Wisconsin. An entire TV series was devoted to the supper club, which is sort of like *Cheers* in that "everybody knows your name." They have a family friendly atmosphere while offering a little more upscale dining—tablecloths and candles. All you have to do is Google "supper clubs" and you'll find books and even a movie about this unique Wisconsin experience. And what would a supper club meal be without the Wisconsin drink: a Brandy Old-Fashioned. Yep. Brandy. I once heard of a Chicago bartender, who, when the patron requested a Brandy Old-Fashioned, said, "You must be from Wisconsin." I long ago crossed supper clubs off of my to-do list. And, like fish fries, I continue to enjoy this unique aspect of Wisconsin.

As far as "big" birds go, central Wisconsin has sandhill cranes, and it has been a delight to see them from "fairly" close and hear their loud call when they fly overhead—they sound like what I imagine elephants gargling sound like. We didn't see sandhills in Milwaukee. Wisconsin has a crane preserve where one can see fifteen types of cranes. I hope to visit soon.

I crossed off the hunting and fishing goal, too, when I attended a "Becoming an Outdoor Woman" weekend, where I took a gun safety class and fired a 12 gauge shotgun at clay pigeons. On that same weekend, I went fly fishing in a river. Our instructor wore pearls and gave us each a string of plastic pearls. She showed us a picture of England's Queen Mother fly fishing in waders and pearls, and said, "If she can do it, we can do it!"

We practiced casting by swooshing the rod from "eleven o'clock" to "one o'clock." Casting is an art, and I didn't master it that day, but I liked trying it for the first time. I didn't catch a trout, but that didn't matter.

I still remember the slippery rocks under my feet and the sensation of cold water flowing around my rubber waders. It's not every day you stand in a river.

But so far I hadn't gone kayaking, and I wondered if my window of opportunity was closing.

Then, I was invited to a cottage weekend with the promise of some kayaking as well.

"Boating," as kayakers say, was everything I hoped it would be.

First, this was *not* the type of kayaking where one "shoots the rapids" and needs prior training about how to escape from a turned-over boat.

This is what we did: four women ages sixty-five to eighty-two transported four kayaks on two small trailer hitches from the cottage to the lake. It took two trips. There was more involved than I realized since the kayaks were firmly strapped to the hitch and needed to be untied and the bungee cords unhooked. Then we carried them down to the water.

Once all four kayaks floated in the shallow water, I sat down in the first one, and Margaret shoved me off of the shore. What a relief when my knees bent enough to get into the kayak. That was the part I was most concerned about.

On this after-supper excursion, we had Little Fox

Lake to ourselves. The next hour left me feeling like a true Wisconsinite as I paddled my way through water lilies closing their yellow petals for the evening. I looked through clear brown water and watched for smooth rocks among the undulating vines and reeds. A couple of cottage-goers sat on lawn chairs by their docks, enjoying the still evening.

Our hostess guided us through a narrow inlet to Newt Pond, where the paddling required a little more skill. I plowed right into a stand of reeds, but, hurrah, I was able to back out and steer to the deeper water. We did not see much wildlife—only a turtle sunning on a log—but we heard birds calling.

I loved the feeling of being on the water, moved by the current and wind. A light breeze carried the rich smell of wet mud and damp vegetation. With my khaki hat pulled over my head, I was immersed in nature, plain and unglamorous, and just where I wanted to be.

After an hour, we returned to our launch point. Getting out of the kayak proved more difficult than getting in, as lake water slicked the boat bottom—but I managed, with an assist from my friends. It must have looked like they were hauling in a beached whale.

Then, the four of us carried the kayaks back to the hitches, which remained untouched by the side of the road, even though occasional cars and pickups passed by. After lifting the boats into place, we tied them and re-stretched the bungee cords. Again, it took two trips to return the kayaks and paddlers back to the cottage. Kayaking wasn't just floating—it took work.

It felt good to have new experiences. I believe it was Yogi Berra who said, "It ain't over 'til it's over."

Chapter 8
Lessons through the Ages

Anna slept over on Monday night. Her mouth hurt a little because the orthodontist had tightened her braces, so I made her macaroni and cheese, applesauce, and fruit cocktail for dinner. She loved it.

Anna wanted to "interview" me, and she typed the questions and my answers on her laptop.

"How did you like growing up with three younger sisters?"

"I didn't like it. I thought they were bratty. I liked them better when they were older."

"I was not expecting you to say that," Anna laughed.

Then we watched a movie she brought—the live-action version of *Cinderella*. At bedtime, she asked me to sing to her. I love singing to her and tucking her hair behind her ear. I sang, "Down by the Station," "Tura Lura," "If You're Good from Day to Day," and "Thank you, God."

Tuesday morning we ate pancakes for breakfast, and

Amanda picked her up at 9:30 a.m.

Wednesday morning, Amanda waved to me as she and Anna and Justin went by on their walk. I saw them through my patio door and waved back.

Wednesday afternoon, Amanda called to see if I wanted to go out for a "three generation dinner" with her and Anna. Justin had to work, and Nate was at camp all week. Amanda picked me up later that afternoon and looked so summery in white pants and a blue top. Anna wore a white sundress and white sandals. Her light brown hair was brushed straight, with one small braid on the side to keep her hair off her face. Her golden necklace spelled "love" in cursive writing.

Amanda said, "We were thinking Mexican, but can't decide where to go." I asked, "What is El Tequila Salsa like? I've never been there." Amanda thought it was a good choice, so off we went.

Tamales with a Corona Light tasted especially good after a spontaneous dinner invitation. Most seniors I knew jumped at a chance to spend time with family.

On Thursday, a big rain storm with heavy winds blew in right around the noon hour. Amanda called to see if I lost power like they had. Nope, my power was still on. "You can come over if you'd like," I offered.

Amanda asked, "Is it okay if I bring the wet clothes in my washing machine over there to dry them?"

"Of course."

So, Thursday afternoon Amanda and Anna came over for a couple of hours. Kneeling on my living room carpet, Anna colored an owl with her markers. She and Amanda split a root beer. Amanda and I chatted about their Toyota they'd put up for sale, Anna's upcoming third-grade year, Nate's camp experience, and how to use various apps on my new smartphone.

When the clothes were dry and folded, I tore the owl page out of the coloring book so Anna could finish at home. Anna clung to me and rested her head on my chest. It was hard to say goodbye.

I wrote this activity down for my writers' group which meets on Wednesdays. Jane said, "Now we know why you moved here." Being part of busy family life was over so soon. That's why we cherish those moments when they happen.

***

We ladies at the "resort" joked that changing the bed linens was enough exercise for the day. And once, I was ambitious enough to wash the mattress pad at the coin laundry we had on-site. Their washing machines were better for bulky items.

Afterward, the freshly-laundered pad curled in the middle of the bed like a fist. I looked at it with my hands on my hips. "I am a college graduate and you are a mattress pad. I am sure we can come to some sort of agreement." No response.

"Okay," I said. "I see you are not going to cooperate. However, I remember from last time your label goes in the lower right corner of the bed. Show me your label." I grabbed the still-warm-from-the-dryer pad and began turning it in my hands, trying to find the label. The pad resisted, but finally I announced, "Aha! I've got you!" I maneuvered that corner of the pad over the mattress.

Carefully, I pulled the pad kitty-corner. It was way too short. I obviously misremembered which corner the label matched. I moved the label to the upper right side of the bed, stre-e-etched the pad out, and the whole thing popped off the corner.

"I see you are determined to be difficult," I growled.

Kneeling on the bed, I tucked the pad in with a vengeance and pulled carefully to the lower left corner. No dice. The pad popped off again.

I stood up straight and looked all around at the walls and ceiling.

"Am I on *Candid Camera*?"

But there was no Allen Funt to shake my hand and say, "Smile!"

Back to the upper right corner. That time, I pulled over to the upper left. Yes! Carefully, I pulled the pad down to the bottom and anchored it. Finally, victory.

The television was full of scary commercials advocating the purchase of a new mattress after seven years. They tell you how your mattress is full of dried skin cells and dust mites.

Once I had a clean mattress pad and fresh sheets, I hated to put my old pillows into the laundered pillow cases. I tossed the pillows in a warm dryer for thirty minutes each. If the heat didn't kill the mites, I hoped the dryer at least made them dizzy.

After all that exertion, I sat in my recliner and put my feet up. No sooner did I sit, when through my patio door I spied Evangeline walking outside on the grass.

Oh my goodness, I thought, as I jumped up and opened the sliding door.

From my patio, I could see Evangeline rapping on my next door neighbor's glass doors. Apparently, Vivian was not home. I walked over to Evangeline and said,"Hi, Evangeline. Can I help you?"

She looked at me, and again said, "I'm looking for the lady—with the windmill . . ."

"I'll help you," I said. "Let's go through my apartment."

She was quite docile, and she followed me over the grass, through my patio doors and apartment, and then we walked through the building to her Cousin Julia's apartment.

It was September, and just the thought of her wandering outside when cold weather sets in is very concerning. I felt I needed to make a call to the office, and they were very kind, thanked me, and said they couldn't say much "due to confidentiality," but they were aware of the problem.

**

Here's another "I can't believe I did that" moment.

This time, as usual, the start was innocent enough. Due to an unexpected cold snap, I decided to cut down my basil. Ultimately, I planned to chop the leaves with some olive oil and freeze the oil/herb mixture in ice cube trays. The branches were so fragrant and bright green that I saved them in a glass of water on my dining room table for a few days. They made a beautiful centerpiece on my blue tablecloth. The ceiling fan wafted the basil aroma around the apartment.

Every day I admired them and thought, "Should I chop those leaves now?" But I decided to wait a bit longer.

On the fourth day, I felt motivated to get out my blender and the extra-virgin olive oil. All went well as I chopped the leaves into the green oil and scraped the rich mixture into ice cube trays. My kitchen smelled of Little Italy, like plump green olives and fresh basil. It would be wonderful to add those cubes to soups or stews this fall.

The bare basil branches were thrown into the trash, the blender disassembled and cleaned, and the counters mopped. Then, I was thirsty, so I drank half a glass of water sitting on the counter.

Moments later, I spied my water glass on the back of the sink. Why were there two water glasses out?

I drank the vase water. One good thing: it didn't taste or smell bad, so the water couldn't have been *too* nasty!

About four hours later, my gut gave me the answer. Cramps and diarrhea set in. *Are you kidding me? I've put bacteria into my body by drinking that water! And now this!"*

A miserable few hours ensued, followed the next day by a diet of soup, bananas, saltines, and beverages with electrolytes.

My friend Joanna from book group called and wanted to go out for lunch. "Not today," I demurred, "but tomorrow I have another 'I can't believe I did that' story for you."

"I can't wait," she said.

***

What can we learn from Emma Morano, the world's

oldest woman, who died recently in Italy?

She was 117 years and 137 days old at the time of her death.

She had not left her apartment since she was 102. That means for more than fifteen years people looked after her and provided for her. Although she lived alone, she was part of a community.

For the last twenty-seven years of her life she lived in a tiny two-room apartment. Who needs more? Tiny houses are coming into vogue in the United States. "Grandma Pods" are playhouse-sized residences the adult children can put in their backyards to have Grandma nearby. In my travels to South America, I saw whole families living in cardboard box cities. It is more than time to return to reasonable living spaces and to provide affordable housing for those just starting out, rather than mega-mansions.

In the 1960s, there was a rule of thumb: buy a house that cost no more than twice your annual income. Somehow, that rule seems to have fallen by the wayside. I like what Calvin Coolidge once said:

"There is no dignity quite so impressive, and no

independence quite so important, as living means."

Charles Dickens, in *David Copperfield*, created a beloved character, Mr. Micawber, whose financial advice is famous:

"Annual income twenty pounds, annual expenditure nineteen pounds, result happiness.

Annual income twenty pounds, annual expenditure twenty-one pounds, result misery."

Emma Morano did not have the stress that often comes with married life or children. She briefly married, but separated in 1938 and said, "Never again." She also had an infant son who was born and died in 1937. Arthur and I agreed to divorce after thirty years of marriage, and for twenty years thereafter we both enjoyed the new lives we created for ourselves. Marriage should be a thoughtful decision, and divorce should remain a thoughtful option.

She worked until she was seventy-five and was proud to support herself. That says a lot about the desire many women have for fulfillment outside the home, as well as the contribution women make to the workforce. If women want to work they need to be able to manage the size of their families. Women, like men, need to be able to follow their own dreams. I know how much I enjoyed my career at an insurance company before I retired.

Until age 112, Emma cooked for herself. Usually pasta. Cooking is so enjoyable. Food is one of the great pleasures of life.

In the last years of her life, her simple clothing consisted of a house dress with a vest or a shawl. We do have too many clothes— way more than we need. Once I retired, my wardrobe was much smaller than it was when I was working. And as the years go on, I'm sure it will shrink further. Have you seen the tiny closets in assisted living apartments? We go from walk-in closets in our old homes to having just enough space for a sweater, a bathrobe, and a second pair of slacks. We will all be like Emma one day.

She was devout, and family pictures decorated her living space. Faith and family. Isn't that what life comes down to? We should all clear our lives of things that don't really matter.

Chapter 9
The Things We Keep

Amanda asked, "Mom, why do you still have that old thing?"

She meant my olive green coffee percolator, which dated back to the 1970s. Remember olive green? Remember percolators? There is a basket for the coffee grounds, and a stem that sends water up over the grounds. It used to make twenty-four cups of coffee and made a satisfying "chug chug" sound while the coffee perked. When the coffee was ready, you stuck your cup under the little black spigot and held the handle to one side to dispense a cupful of coffee.

At some point, the water quit rising up the stem, so the percolator no longer "perks." Why did I hold onto it then?

Every fall I dragged it out from the back of the cupboard because it was perfect to make hot cider for a group. It heated a half-gallon of apple pressings to the perfect temperature. I hung a tea ball in the pot with cloves and allspice and added one or two sticks of cinnamon. A little orange juice and concentrated lemonade completed the delicious hot drink—much better than those packets of apple cider mix from the store.

When my friends arrived for book club or bridge, they always said, "Mmmm, it smells so good in here." The aroma of apple cider and cinnamon is simply one of the best parts of autumn.

Which is why I can't bring myself to get rid of the olive green percolator. Maybe I will invite my new writers' group to visit my apartment, and I'll serve hot cider and oatmeal cake. Then the percolator will go in the back of the cupboard until next year.

Recipe for "Hot Spiced Cider"
One gallon apple cider
½ t. salt
36 whole cloves
12 whole allspice
1 four-inch cinnamon stick
¼ c. sugar
¼ c. frozen orange juice concentrate
2 Tablespoons frozen lemonade concentrate

Heat first six ingredients, but do not boil. Stir in orange and lemonade concentrate. If desired, decorate each mug with a thin quarter of an orange slice with a clove stuck in it. Makes sixteen one-cup servings.

***

I also kept an antique iron, used as a bookend. It's the cordless, cast iron type that must weigh five pounds. Great Grandmother probably heated it on the back of her wood burning stove. The antique iron was decorative, and my electric iron was hardly used either. This week I walked past another apartment and saw freshly-ironed blouses on the door hanger. One of the other residents must have done some ironing for another resident. What a generous soul.

I began to reminisce about ironing.

In the 1950s, Monday was wash day and most of the day Tuesday was spent ironing. Mother told me she enjoyed ironing. She "sprinkled" the clothes and sheets with water, rolled them in a ball, and piled them on the end of the ironing board. The sprinkling and "rest" time dampened the article all the way through, making it easier to press out the wrinkles. Other mothers I knew put the rolled items in the refrigerator until it was their turn to be ironed. Mother taught me how to iron pillowcases and my dad's handkerchiefs. I loved inhaling the smell of those freshly-ironed pillowcases—a heady scent of heat and fresh air from the outdoor clothesline that no one has been able to bottle. It was fun to iron handkerchiefs. I folded them in half and then in half again, and piled the neatly pressed little squares in a tall tower.

To determine if the iron was hot enough, you wet your finger in your mouth and then touched the iron—quickly. The loud hissing told you the iron was ready. If you were too slow about it, you burned your finger. You also could sprinkle some water on the ironing board and test the iron that way, but that didn't have the element of danger. Either way gave you the satisfying "sssssss" sound.

We were fortunate to own a wringer washing machine. No one had dryers in those days. Clothes dried outside on the clothesline or in the basement on rainy days which made roller skating around the furnace difficult as we dodged the damp sheets hanging in our path.

In those days, almost everything got ironed. "Pants pressers" were long wire inserts put into damp jeans fresh from the washer. The pants dried into a stiff, smooth, board-like pair, but it was one less item to iron.

Some homes built in the 1950s had a designated ironing board closet in the kitchen where you opened the door and folded down a wooden ironing board. The house we bought in the 1970s had one of those, but the ironing board had been removed and shelves added, converting the closet to a spice rack.

In the 1960s, clothes dryers became more prevalent, and "permanent press" came along, but ironing continued. At my college, every dormitory floor had an ironing board and iron. A friend showed me how to iron a gathered skirt, working the point of the iron up into the gathers, yet ironing the skirt part smooth. My boyfriend's sister taught me how to iron a man's shirt. She proudly stated she "could iron a shirt in four minutes." First the collars and cuffs, then the shoulder yoke, followed by the button and buttonhole facings. Last of all, the broader expanses of the sides and back.

Mother gave me a Sunbeam iron for a wedding present.

It was a steam iron with a blue cloth-covered electric cord (so much more elegant than a plain black cord) and a little receptacle at the top for water. For a spurt of steam, you just pressed a button at the top of the iron. The instructions advised using distilled water to avoid buildup of minerals in the iron, but I used plain water. For me, ironing was done out of necessity. Some of my peers, however, ironed sheets and even their husband's underwear. They were the same women who vacuumed and dusted every day.

In the late '60s and early '70s, the Vietnam war was a big part of our lives. Arthur attended Officer Candidate School in Fort Sill, Oklahoma, and the Candidates' wives starched and ironed their husbands' uniforms. We often wondered how an unmarried officer candidate managed without someone pressing his fatigues for him. A big part of our daily routine was picking up the used fatigues or khakis and dropping off the stiffly starched and pressed set. Another activity of the military wives was making red fireproof curtains for the barracks. (The senior candidates were called Redbirds—hence the red curtains.) We made the fabric flame-retardant using a solution of water and 20 Mule Team Borax. Of course, after the curtains had been washed in this solution, we ironed them.

Fire in the barracks should have been the least of our worries when our husbands were being trained to "call in" artillery fire in a jungle. But the ordinary tasks kept our minds off of what was actually happening.

By the '80s, the ironing board had a permanent place in our bedroom. I starched Arthur's shirts in the laundry and then ironed a fresh one for him every morning. The iron also pressed out any wrinkles behind the knees of his dress pants before he set out for the day. The iron served our two children, too. There were "iron on" patches for the knees of Alan's pants. They didn't adhere that well; a corner always seemed to curl up. I sewed dresses for Amanda, which meant pressing seams flat and ironing puffy sleeves and skirts.

The iron pressed autumn leaves between sheets of wax paper for Brownie and Cub Scout crafts. An "ironing bag" held items that could wait for attention, like cloth napkins and aprons. In those busy years, if something got added to the ironing bag, it waited a long time before being brought out again.

The Christmas when Amanda was six, she proudly gave me a new ironing board cover. She and I were both sincerely thrilled. It really freshened up the old board.

Of course, there were some ironing disasters. The new nylon/rayon/acetate fabrics and irons were not meant to go together. If the iron was hot, those fabrics melted right on the iron, with a scorched chemical smell. It was not easy cleaning melted nylon off an iron, and the imprint of an iron on those fabrics meant the article was ruined forever. If the tip of the iron came too close to your fingers on a pointed collar or a triangular dart, you would soon feel the stinging burn, and a tiny blister reminded you to take more care.

I once sprayed a shirt with spray starch and ran the iron over the white foam. There was a terrible smell, though, and the odor stayed in the shirt. Too late I realized the aerosol can was not spray starch—it contained pre-wash stain remover. That shirt had to go through the wash again. It came out nice and clean, though.

In the '90s I went to work full-time. Arthur sent his shirts out to the laundry. The kids became young adults and were off in college or apartments. I visited my son at school and ironed some of his shirts. I seldom ironed for myself—only if absolutely necessary. New fabrics meant ironing was often not needed, especially if you grabbed something out of the dryer quickly enough. I got rid of the ironing bag and cloth napkins. I learned to "smooth" T-shirts with my hands; they almost looked ironed.

Recently, I conducted an informal survey to learn about ironing in the twenty-first century.

"Do you iron?" I asked the employees at my credit union.

"No."

"Never."

"Only if I have to."

"If the clothes come out of the dryer wrinkled, I throw them back in the dryer for a while and then they're okay."

"My mother-in-law does—she irons everything!"

"Do you own an iron?"

"Yes." They all agreed that they did.

"How about an ironing board?"

"Yes," to that as well.

"It's in the basement somewhere."

One woman actually owns two ironing boards—the tabletop variety as well as the fold-up kind. She seldom uses them, though.

Living in my "senior" apartment, I have rediscovered ironing—blouses look so nice with the crease in the sleeve. Ironing seemed almost pleasurable again, the way the wrinkles responded to your bidding and gave way to smooth flatness. There was a quilting group here, and they pressed every square, block, and seam. Bonnie did tailoring for the other residents. (She replaced the zipper in my winter coat.) She always had the ironing board up in her living room.

In a fast changing world, it was surprising to look back and see the iron as a way of recalling the phases of life. There were times I ironed daily, and there were times I ignored the iron completely. Those I surveyed may not iron now, but perhaps they will later. And, if nothing else, they will have a good bookend, like my antique iron.

***

I couldn't catch myself.

My right knee hit the floor first. Next, both hands skidded across the carpet. Finally, the left side of my face slammed into the ground, and my glasses flew two feet across the hallway.

As I lay in the hall at Bentwood, I knew nothing was broken, thank goodness. My new slippers had tripped me up again. I bought the fuzzy, gray slide-ons last month and had stumbled over them several times. Today my luck ran out. I was going along at a pretty good clip and could not save myself from a fall.

You knew this was going to happen—but, no, you thought you would adjust to this slipper style. Amanda will say, "Mom, you should always take your cell phone with you."

I craned my neck and couldn't believe my good fortune—no one had seen me take a header. "Well, I was just walking to the mailroom—" sounded pretty lame.

My activity didn't go completely unnoticed, however. GiGi, Pauline's little Yorkshire terrier, was having a complete fit, barking behind the apartment door closest to me. I heard Pauline scolding, "Stop barking, Gigi."

I managed to return to a sitting position. Any minute

Pauline would open the door to see what upset GiGi so much. I could just imagine Pauline saying, "My goodness, Nancy! Are you all right?" She probably wasn't accustomed to seeing a resident sitting on the floor.

Gigi, the little brown and blonde dog, would scamper around me in the hall.

I turned to crouch on all fours and then stood. I picked up my glasses from the floor. One stem was a little bent out of shape. So far, there was no major damage except for a rug burn on my thumb that was bleeding.

I held my hand aloft and limped down the hall toward my door. Yes, I was smart enough to carry the offending slippers under my arm.

These are going to Goodwill—they tripped me up for the last time.

When I fell in the snow, no one knew about it but me. Here, I could keep it a secret if no little dogs were out and about. But someone was sure to come along. I was not alone.

Chapter 10
Special Dinners and Taco Tuesday

Bentwood Hills hosted another luncheon. The rodeo-themed menu included sloppy joes, baked beans, carrot sticks, and apple pie for dessert. They offered lemonade and coffee to drink.

Evangeline took the empty chair next to me. Perhaps she felt she knew me since she had wandered into my apartment so many times. Inwardly, I rolled my eyes. Where was that husband of hers, anyway? According to the grapevine, after Evangeline got lost going to Bingo, management asked him to accompany her at all times.

I looked around and spotted him sitting alone next to a large potted rubber plant. Was he keeping an eye on her from that vantage point, or was he lurking there to avoid helping her? I glanced at Evangeline's place and noticed she had the cream pitcher from the coffee area. She poured the entire pitcher of cream into her cup. I asked her, "Evangeline, do you want some coffee?"

"No," she replied. "I want milk."

Well, that wasn't milk, but no matter.

When we were almost finished eating, Evangeline said, "I want coffee."

"Let me go with you," I said. Together, we walked over to the beverage table and I helped her with the coffee pot, sugar, and Styrofoam cups. The cream pitcher was back at her place, of course. There was no way she could manage on her own, as she did not remember how to put her cup under the spigot and hold it down. Plus, her balance was shaky.

Meanwhile, her husband sat by the plant and twiddled his thumbs.

Speaking of coffee, Bentwood Hills always used to have the coffee pot on, and a resident could stop in the community room any time during the day to have a cup and visit with other people. Unfortunately, Bentwood discontinued the bottomless cup because some people took advantage of it. One resident brought his thermos down and filled it to take back to his apartment. Now that was cheap.

Another time, Maxine and Harold reserved the community room for their fiftieth anniversary party.

Afterward, Maxine was cleaning up and making trips back to her apartment. She took a load of serving dishes and admitted that she did "putter" for a few minutes, but not long. When she returned to the community kitchen for the rest of her things, she found someone had taken the remaining half of their anniversary cake!

In addition to enjoying activities at Bentwood, this past fall I started volunteering at a local elementary school. They had a "homework club" after school for their English language learners, who were Hmong. The children were adorable. They all spoke English very well, but they needed enrichment. Many did not speak English at home.

Working with these children reminded me how complicated the English language can be. The third graders read to me one-on-one, and I asked them questions to make sure they comprehended what they were reading. We read a book about "Freddy the Turtle," in which Freddy went into the "cloakroom" at his school. I doubted if my granddaughter Anna knew what a cloakroom was, so I especially doubted a child of Hmong origin knew.

Another time we read an *Amelia Bedelia* book. Amelia was very literal and was always getting mixed up. We read about how Amelia's employer asked her to plant bulbs in the garden. Well, she planted light bulbs. That led to a good discussion about how the same word can have different meanings.

Then, in the same story, Amelia's employer asked her to ice some cupcakes. And the man of the house came home from a fishing trip with his catch and asked Amelia to ice his fish. The little girl who was reading to me knew what ice was, but she did not know "frosting" can also be called "icing." So she expected Amelia to put ice on the cupcakes. Silly Amelia, she put frosting on the fish.

It was fun to spend time with the children once a week and to help them improve their English.

One night, I played bridge in the library, as I do every week. The library was also the place where the post office and UPS dropped off packages that didn't fit in our little mailboxes. Well, we were playing cards, and Dorothy walked in wearing her long turquoise bathrobe that zipped up the front. "Don't look at me, you all," she had said. "I just remembered I got a package, and

I couldn't wait until tomorrow to pick it up. It has the candy I ordered."

We all had a good laugh. There was something about residents wandering into the library in their bathrobe that felt like family.

Between the Hmong children and the informal residents in my building, I felt more at home in this new town.

***

Bentwood Hills had a social group to plan activities for the residents in addition to the ones organized by management. The social group organized day trips and potluck suppers. I volunteered to plan "Taco Tuesday."

Seventy people made reservations, and many volunteered to bring a dessert and/or help with preparations. The local butcher gave us a discount on fifteen pounds of ground chuck. We spent $100.76 at Aldi's for lettuce, tomatoes, refried beans, guacamole, cheddar cheese, sour cream, black olives, tortillas, tomatoes, onions, and taco seasoning. It makes my mouth water just remembering those yummy ingredients.

We charged three dollars per person and each received two tacos—plus, the selection of desserts was amazing. Barbara made individual crème brulees in little ramekins. That was really over the top. There were also brownies, carrot cake, blueberry cheesecake, and the ever-popular lemon bars. It seemed everyone wanted to try a little bit of each.

The committee gathered in the afternoon to do all of the cooking and prep work as well as set the tables. We nominated Richard for the lucky job of chopping onions. We were happy to let him do it. Trudy lent us her handy-dandy onion chopper that diced the onion in one fell swoop. The aroma of chopped onions was overwhelming. And there was something about bustling around the kitchen together that felt companionable.

Trudy volunteered to wrap plastic forks and spoons in paper napkins. She took the forks, spoons, and napkins to her apartment so she could work on them at her dining room table. Mildred told me later that she sat at the table and drank a cup of coffee while Trudy wrapped.

Trudy wasn't sure how many residents would attend the potluck, so she wrapped 100 sets. Mildred said, "I asked her, 'Don't you ever listen to your messages? Your message light is blinking.'"

So Trudy listened to three messages on her answering machine. One message said seventy residents had signed up for the dinner.

According to Mildred, Trudy then counted out seventy wrapped forks and carefully unwrapped the remaining thirty. She got out her ironing board and began to iron the thirty paper napkins since they had curled.

Mildred said she watched her for a moment, and then she admitted, "I kind of barked at her."

Mildred said to Trudy, "Why didn't you just leave them wrapped for the next dinner?"

"I didn't think about that," Trudy admitted.

She carefully stacked the ironed paper napkins and brought them back down to the community kitchen while Mildred rolled her eyes.

Folks started wandering in as early as 3:30 p.m., commenting, "It sure smells good!"

All you have to do is chop an onion and the kitchen smells good. Then, brown some ground chuck and everyone's mouth starts watering. By 4:30 p.m., guests were putting on their name tags and finding a place at the tables to sit and visit until we served at 5:00 p.m. Joanna acted as a greeter. We always had a few new people, and it was nice to have someone help them find a seat.

I noticed that old people liked to be early birds. And I was one of them. I didn't like to be rushed or miss a good seat.

The event was a success, with a little money left over for next month. One man called as he left, "You folks did a great job, as always."

Larry and June always volunteered for cleanup, and they did a much-appreciated job. We used paper plates and plastic utensils, but there was still the Nesco to scrub and all of the serving bowls.

Some refried beans were left over. When we served, a few folks said, "I'll pass on those." Dee ladled the beans, and she had said, "I'm starting to feel a bit rejected over here." I recommend that we buy less next time.

It was just another reason to enjoy life at Bentwood Hills—great food and camaraderie.

Chapter 11
Senior Moments

A credit union offered a day trip for their customers aged fifty and over as a marketing technique for their business. Joanna and I enjoyed the all-day Fall Color Tour—a bus ride to Eagle River, three hours at Cranberry Fest, a bus ride to Rhinelander and then a two-hour dinner cruise on the Wisconsin River before busing back to Westown—all for sixty-five dollars per person.

We were supposed to depart from an insurance company parking lot at 9:00 a.m. We arrived at 8:35 and were not the first ones—other early birds were already waiting. The Lamers bus arrived and the driver incorrectly drove into the lot next door—a medical facility parking area. Soon, cars formed a line driving over there. Then, the credit union organizer started waving us all back to the insurance company lot, and we followed each other like lemmings.

It was like that all day. Everyone was in a hurry to be first in line, even if it meant standing and waiting. First in line for the bus, first in line for the boat ride, first on top of the upper deck, first in line for dinner. I didn't know if that was a senior citizen characteristic or just human nature. Joanna and I were perfectly satisfied with our seat toward the middle of the bus.

We could not have asked for a more beautiful day—sunny and sixty-eight degrees. Cranberry Fest was known all around Wisconsin. I was happy to cross another Wisconsin experience off of my bucket list—I found that seniors really enjoyed day trips. There were no worries about driving or parking. Our social committee at Bentwood organized a couple of day trips last summer and they were well attended. They even went on an all-day trip to Milwaukee to a Brewers game at Miller Park.

The Cranberry Fest grounds covered about an acre, with artist and vendor tents set up in orderly rows. There was a model cranberry bog, but somehow we missed that. I bought cranberry cheddar cheese, cranberry-jalapeño mustard, cranberry jam, some cranberry dried snack mix, and cranberry jelly beans. Some items could be Christmas gifts.

Seniors might not be a good market for most fest

merchandise unless it was food-related. We no longer needed the lovely garden décor, hand-thrown pottery bowls and coffee mugs, large watercolor paintings, or even the North Woods-look furniture with black bears on the throw pillows—we were past all that and into the downsizing phase of life.

I looked for a one-of-a-kind embroidered jeans jacket but didn't see anything in my style. Everything was bedazzled. I definitely wasn't the rhinestone type.

We drank lemonade and people-watched for the last hour. With the impending presidential election, we avoided those who obnoxiously displayed their choices on their heads or their backs. Seeing our chaperones at the park entrance, we walked over to inquire if the bus had arrived. It was just down the street. "He has his door open; you can go ahead and board," we were told. Guess what? We were the first ones back. Maybe I missed the ideal jeans jacket, but I got to sit in the comfy bus before the other tired seniors straggled onboard.

On the river cruise, we saw an eagle sitting high in a tree—it was hard not to imagine him as a protector surveying our comings and goings. Later, we saw the giant nest of an eagle or osprey, built out of uncomfortable-looking sticks. I have no idea how these birds make such intricate nests, but sometimes we sacrifice comfort for sturdiness. That nest would certainly withstand Wisconsin winds.

We basked in the light breeze from the upper deck of the boat. From this vantage point, we saw why this was called the Fall Color Tour. Orange and red splashes on the serene brown surface of the river mirrored the landscape. One man next to us had his camera out. I wondered if people were so busy taking pictures that they missed seeing life's gifts with their own eyes. I tried to stay in the moment and enjoy the beauty, not thinking about what else fall meant—winter was on the way.

Our companions at dinner talked about some of the day trips they had taken. They especially enjoyed the casino trips. The gentleman had warm brown eyes and a blue baseball cap. One front tooth protruded longer than the other, and as he spoke, the extended tooth waggled loosely back and forth. I restrained myself from nodding my head in time with his tooth.

"You need to put your money in different banks," he

advised. "Then you are on more mailing lists for these trips."

***

I flew to North Carolina for a few days' visit with my sister Sandra and her husband Rich. That was my first trip since moving from my own home into an apartment. How easy to lock the door behind me and leave worry-free about my apartment—I didn't even set any lights on timers to "make it look like someone was home." Marie, my neighbor, would pick up the daily newspaper we shared and watch for any packages. Leaving the apartment was the simplest part of my trip. Airports, with all of their security and restrictions, were not the fun they used to be, so I was a little stressed about making my connections, having the correct-sized quart plastic bag for liquids, parking, etc.

I needed to leave at 5:00 in the morning. Amanda offered to take me to the airport, but I knew she had to get the kids off to school. A couple of my friends from Bentwood said they would be happy to drive me, but I felt that the early hour would be an imposition. Therefore, I drove myself and parked where my daughter suggested. I breezed through security because I was "TSA Pre-checked," although I did not know it. I didn't have to take off my shoes, show my liquids, etc. That was a relief.

At the gate, I took advantage of early boarding "for those who needed a little extra time." "Come on up," the attendant told me. "Don't be shy." She gate-checked my bag and put the claim ticket on for me. I was glad. Those twisty bands on claim tickets were confusing. I must have looked like I needed help. And you know I liked to get on *early* to get settled.

In my cramped aisle seat on the plane, I dropped magazine subscription offers out of *People* and onto the floor. I also knocked my so-called "cookie" off of the tray table and into the aisle. Was I three years old? I used to be more coordinated. My excuse was you could hardly move your elbows in those seats.

My connection was through Detroit Airport which has an underground tunnel with walkway belts. I moved to the right so someone could pass me and careened into the rail. Balance was not my strong point, particularly on moving walkways. Luckily, my carry-on bag kept me from falling over. The lady behind me asked, "Are you okay?" I tried to reassure her with a hearty "I'm fine." Like most people, I didn't want any fuss and acted pluckier than I really felt.

To get to concourse "A," there was an escalator or an elevator. *Hmmmm*. I opted for the elevator. Me going *down* an escalator with a suitcase? Not a pretty picture.

With a three-hour layover in Detroit, and feeling a bit like a rickety old person, I decided to splurge on a ten-minute chair massage. "Steven" found knots I didn't know I had.

When I went to pay, he surprised me with a request to scan my boarding pass. I asked why, and he explained the airport had my ID information from the pass, so the massage business did not need to ask for ID. Also, after a massage, people were a little loopy and tended to forget things. By scanning the boarding pass, they had the gate number and could return lost items. Interesting.

I purchased a pastry next door at Starbucks for my lunch on the plane. When I came out and tried to read a sign, my vision was blurry. Yep. I left my glasses on the chair at the massage place.

Sure enough, Steven came huffing and puffing with my glasses. The dear soul went to my gate first and then came running back to find me.

Sigh. With only forty minutes to boarding, I decided to sit with my *New York Times* and not cause trouble. Airports were great for people watching.

Why do some women fuss? I noticed a middle-aged couple. He had a neat gray beard and a black beret. His stylish wife wore a long shirt and black newsboy hat. While he ignored her and read, she could not stop fussing—standing over the waiting room seat, moving objects from one carry-on to another, putting her Bible in an outside pocket, zipping and unzipping, making a cell call, snapping the phone shut, taking out a sweatshirt. All the while, she frowned and muttered. Her husband let her fuss. Then, as boarding was called, he smiled gently at her with tired eyes, and they joined the line together.

There weren't many passengers who appeared as old as I was. It was amazing how everyone becomes younger than you. It was also difficult to conceptualize my own age. For example, I still thought I looked like I was in my fifties. In reality, I probably looked a little older than I actually was—more like mid seventies. I was now the "little old lady" who was flying—very weird. Everyone around me was younger. Even other white-haired folks were probably in their late forties to fifties. I reminded myself of the saying, "Don't worry about old age—it doesn't last long."

The woman wearing a ball cap saying "Life is Good?" I have yet to see her stop frowning.

In addition to people watching, I eavesdropped a little. Two ladies sitting next to me had an interesting conversation.

The lady said to her friend, "I have learned a lot since I started working at the eye doctor's office. This week we had a lady in who was complaining that her eyes were stinging. We asked her if she had tried changing her saline solution for her contacts, but she didn't think that was the problem. Then she said, 'Do you think it's because I use a Sharpie for eyeliner?'"

Oh. My. Goodness.

I couldn't wait to tell that story to Sandra when I saw her. We had a great visit and, thankfully, the return home was uneventful. I even remembered where my car was parked in the parking lot.

Chapter 12
Technology Woes

I took my car in for an oil change and mentioned the electronic passenger windows did not work. Could it be related to the new battery I got last month? Maybe a fuse?

Mike was very kind and showed me there was a button on the door that prevented those windows from being rolled up and down. It was a security feature for parents, apparently. I must have pressed it by accident.

Oh, boy. What a dunce.

Technology was not my strong suit. Even though I used a computer quite a bit, installing a new printer was daunting. And the first time the ink cartridges needed to be changed I thought I might have a heart attack.

Other older people were also technology-challenged. One of my friends told me she didn't want to get a new car because she didn't want to learn the dashboard again. That was the truth. Just figuring out how the windshield wipers and high beams work was enough, let alone the GPS, backup camera, CD player and how to adjust the clock at daylight savings time.

On occasion, I had to call the cable company. Nightmare. At least by then I could tell the difference between the modem—provided by the cable company— and the router, purchased by me. The router provided Wi-Fi in every room in the apartment. I thought.

The cable company always wanted you to get down on your hands and knees and check the connections. Yikes. He didn't know I was a candidate for knee replacement. And there were so many wires. The cable guy was at Bentwood Hills on pretty much a daily basis. And we even got expanded cable included in our rent, so you wouldn't think he would be needed that much.

Last year the cable company went digital, and we all got digital boxes that had our apartment numbers and a skull and crossbones that told us we would walk the plank if we even *thought* about taking it with us when we moved.

The residents were confused about the difference between digital and High Definition, so some thought we would be able to get the HD channels. Wrong. It was all very confusing.

One of my friends took her car into the shop to complain about a humming noise from the back of the car. It turned out that her rear speakers were on.

***

I got a call from Diane, the daughter of my eighty-year-old friend, Laverne. "I haven't been able to get hold of my mother for two days." At some point in the past, Laverne gave Diane my phone number, and she was calling me with concern. Living two hours away, her daily phone contact with her mom was an important ritual.

"Well, several people lost their landlines in the storm we had a couple days ago," I reassured her. "I think I saw her yesterday, but if you like, I can go check on her. We live on the same floor—she's just at the end of the hall."

"I would really appreciate that," Diane said. She gave me permission to go into Laverne's apartment if needed.

As "independent" seniors, we don't have a nurse on staff. We all look out for each other, though.

Before I panicked about Laverne, I decided to check

the underground parking and see if she was home. Sure enough, her cream-colored boat of an Oldsmobile was in its parking space. *She must be home.*

Next, I pounded on her door. When she didn't answer, I knocked on Marie's door across the hall.

"Have you seen Laverne? This isn't her bridge group day—She has to be in there."

After rapping several more times, we called the office. They verified we had family authorization, and then Nina from housekeeping came with the key. We went in and began calling, "Laverne! Maintenance! Laverne!"

Since we usually gathered in our common areas, we didn't typically go into each other's apartments, and certainly not without being invited. But the circumstances seemed to indicate that we needed to be bold.

Everything looked fine in Laverne's dining room. Nina and I glanced at each other and then continued into the living room. It was as neat as a pin, just like Laverne. Next was her bedroom door, which stood open.

We shivered when we peeked into her bedroom. Nothing on the floor. Nina stepped ahead of me, looked back, and said, "She's in bed."

I took a step forward and saw her lying in bed, a rounded lump under her white coverlet.

We rapped on her bedroom door. No response.

We rushed into the bedroom, calling "Laverne! Laverne!" She lay on her side, looking serene, both hands tucked under one ear. I reached out and touched her side, gently, and with a pat called her name again. Nothing. I began to pat with more vigor, continuing to say her name.

Nina said, "I'm calling 911," as she took out her phone.

Just then we heard a gentle snore. Thank goodness. We knew she was alive if we could just wake her up.

More patting, more calling, and finally, she opened her eyes. Of course, we were afraid she would be startled at the sight of us, but she was okay. She looked at us and knew who we were.

"What's wrong?" she asked.

"Sorry to wake you up like this, Laverne. We've been knocking and calling your name. Your daughter is worried about you."

"Well, I was up late watching Stephen Colbert and then I didn't get to sleep until late. What time is it, anyway?

Almost 10:00? Well, I'm a sound sleeper." She sat up and swung her legs over the side of the bed.

Note to self: get some cute, blue, cotton shortie pajamas like Laverne's, in case I am ever awakened in a similar manner. She looked adorable. Her hair wasn't even messed up.

After verifying her landline was still dead, Laverne declared, "I'm going to go buy a Trac Phone." She used to have a cell phone, but it died and she never replaced it.

Laverne called her daughter on my cell and then said goodbye to us. She was ready to get dressed and go buy a phone.

Nina and I left the apartment laughing with relief. "Can you believe what a sound sleeper she is?"

Laverne came to my apartment not long after her purchase, and we settled in to activate her phone online. The "quick start" instructions said she would need her phone ID number and the pin number she had been given. After sorting through five different pamphlets, we located the information we needed and got the phone activated.

However, the phone displayed a message that she

could only make emergency calls because the SIM card was not found. What? Was that like the card in a digital camera? Where was it?

This meant we had to call the customer service number and enter Laverne's new phone number. The voice told us we would have an eight-minute wait and suggested it would call us back at our number if that was more convenient. Duh. The new phone did not send or receive calls, so that wouldn't work.

I put my cell phone on speaker while we waited.

"What's that noise?" Laverne asked.

"I'm on hold," I explained.

"Is that supposed to be music while you wait? It sounds like pans clanging together."

"I know," I agreed. I took it off speaker.

"I can tell I don't like this new phone already," Laverne said. "I like a phone that folds shut. This fool thing is going to be turning itself on when I don't want it on." Yep. We discussed buying a case for it.

"That's how they get your money. If they made a phone that closed you wouldn't need a case." Yep.

Once the nice lady came on the line, I almost felt sorry

for her, having to deal with the blind leading the blind. First, she verified the phone number we just activated.

"Please turn off the phone, and turn it on again." Of course. This was the time-honored solution for all computer problems. But the "Missing SIM Card" message still displayed.

Then, "Please take off the back of the phone, and remove the battery so I can verify if the SIM card is placed correctly."

I thought you were never supposed to remove the back from a phone, but I managed to do as she directed. The battery was a funny, oblong thing, unlike any battery I had ever seen. I lifted it out carefully.

There was nothing underneath the battery. Just one little white rectangle of tape and another piece of tape with the phone ID info.

"Please remove the SIM card."

"There is no card. Just the two rectangles of tape."

"The white rectangle is the SIM card."

"You have got to be kidding. There is no way I can lift that up and replace it."

This went on for a while. She was a very patient lady, I

will say. I prevailed in this case. I knew the phone would be ruined if I lifted the white rectangle. Even after I gently prodded each corner, it showed no signs of removability.

I carefully replaced the battery, lining up the coppery-anode-thingies. I'm not sure if those were lined up before. Maybe that was the problem.

After replacing the back on the phone, we turned it off and then on again. Lo and behold, the SIM Card message disappeared. We then placed a call to my cell phone, and the nice lady also called the Trac phone from the call center.

Once those two calls were successful, she said, "All of our transactions have now been completed." Remember when they used to say, "Is there anything else I can help you with?" Can't say I blamed her, but I didn't let her off the hook that easily.

"Please show me how to set up voicemail," I said.

"Of course, ma'am." We went through those steps.

This time when she said, "All of our transactions have now been completed," I let her go, imagining her running screaming out of the call center to the nearest bar. Laverne and I were ready to join her.

"Well, your phone works, and I set up your voice mailbox," I said to Laverne.

"What's that?" she asked.

There is one more problem. We made an outgoing call, but when we practiced incoming calls neither of us had the right finger pressure to answer the call. We tried stabbing, jabbing, and just using a fingernail, but the darn thing kept ringing.

Oh, well, the call will go to voicemail. And the landline was supposed to be repaired the next day.

Chapter 13
Aging Is Not for the Faint of Heart

Lunch with women in their eighties and nineties was interesting. Were they opinionated? Set in their ways? Facing the world bravely but with physical ailments? Try all of the above.

Five of us went out every other month. Three were from Bentwood Hills and two lived elsewhere. I thought they invited me to join them because I was able to drive on the freeway. Two of them didn't drive at all anymore. This month we selected an Italian restaurant.

Happily, we arrived at the same time, in two cars, and walked into the restaurant together. Not like the time one carload got lost. A hostess ushered us to a table, and immediately Roberta exclaimed, pointing to the ceiling, "This has got to go!" She referred to the surround-sound music system through which an Italian tenor sang opera tunes. The waitress was very willing to accommodate.

"I can turn that music down right away."

Lois turned to me, "Didn't Nancy come?" she demanded.

"I am Nancy," I answered, in what I hoped were mellow tones.

"Oh," she blinked. "Yes, you are. I mean, didn't Vivian come?"

Vivian drove and walked in with us, but she stopped briefly to hang her coat in the vestibule. Soon she joined us—crisis averted.

"Could they make the print on these menus any smaller?"

"I have macular, and I can't read it even with my magnifying glass."

"Why do they have so many words you can't pronounce, like *pepperoncini* and *prosciutto*?"

"Well, you wanted to come to an Italian restaurant," I observed, in what I hoped were still mellow tones as I became aware of a tic in my right eye.

"No, we didn't. We just wanted to try the new lunch at Giovanni's."

I stood corrected.

Selections were made after discussion of all the entrées and prices. I ordered the chicken chili and salad.

Mary commented, "I don't dare try their chicken chili. If it was my own chili, I would know what spices were in it, but I can't trust theirs."

Vivian was also brave enough to order the chicken chili in addition to her Panini entrée.

Vivian's chili was brought to her as an appetizer. Lois was all over that. "Wait a minute. Didn't you have the chili, too?" She wanted to be sure everything was delivered properly.

"I am having my chili with my salad," I observed, in what I doubted was a mellow tone between the grinding of my back teeth.

While we waited, Lois counted the other diners. "Well, if they were hoping to make this a lunch place it won't last long. They'll be going back to dinners only. Hmmph. What are there? Ten people in this place?"

Meanwhile, Roberta regaled us with the story of a man at her complex who actually said to a female resident, "I bet you would look good in the nude." He also delivered their morning newspapers to their doors, and, would you believe it, hinted that he expected a tip. He was stealing her TV Guide, so she solved that problem by having it mailed to her.

"I tip the woman who delivers newspapers in our complex," I observed, in what I knew was a not-so-mellow tone, and I felt bile rising in my stomach.

"Well, we don't! I guess we are just cheap!"

Thankfully, our meals arrived, to choruses of, "Look at the size of that," "Who can get their mouth around that," and "I can never eat all that."

After a few bites of salad, Lois asked me, "What do you think of the salad? I think it's tasteless."

"I like it," I observed in a snappy tone that was definitely no longer mellow. "Look at all the black olives."

Meals finished and take-out boxes in hand, we set our next lunch date for two months from then. I could hardly wait.

"These chairs don't slide on this carpet," Lois struggled. We bundled up to make our getaway, and Vivian squirmed, "I hate wearing scarves, but this wool coat scratches my neck."

Those women were certainly indomitable. I'd be right with them before I knew it. I aged ten years in their company.

Chapter 14
It's All Downhill: Thoughts on Death and the Afterlife

Last fall I started taking water exercise classes at the Y near here, and I really enjoyed it. The water was very pleasant—it was room temperature. Since I started the class, the range of motion in my right hip improved. Some of the ladies had been attending for years. Two days a week they used Styrofoam weights, and one day was for Styrofoam noodles.

I remember my mother saying that aging was, "Patch! Patch! Patch!" as one thing after another started to go haywire. Louise, a fellow bridge player, started using a walker last fall. She hated to do it, but she had fallen, and the doctor recommended she make the move.

When I was younger, I thought older people went to the doctor frequently out of boredom and loneliness. Now, I understand the body doesn't usually "give out" all at once unless you have a massive heart attack or brain stroke, but rather, things fall apart little by little.

There are phases of life no one can explain to you— you just have to experience them yourself. For example, motherhood. Even if you were the type who wasn't a baby lover, holding your own baby was life changing. No one could explain it to you until it happened.

In the same way, no one could explain what it felt like to grow old. Young people can't imagine that they will ever be old. And that was normal. When I was sixteen, I couldn't imagine myself as an old person, either.

There was a lot to think about as we aged. We wanted to age gracefully, whatever that meant. I think it meant being able to let go of the things of youth like high heels, yet still being engaged in life and learning new things. It's about being the best "you" at whatever age you were. For continued learning, I like "The Great Courses." I purchased college lectures on DVD about Confucius, Greek tragedies, and the Transcendentalist movement. You could also purchase audio tape versions, which were great for long trips in the car.

And, of course, older people began to recognize their mortality, whereas younger people didn't even think about it at all. In my book club, we read *Being*

Mortal, by Dr. Atul Gawande. It was helpful to see that people's needs as they age were not all the same. To some people, it was important to stay in their own home. One of my friends said, "I told myself I would never live somewhere with a number on the door." Others, like me, wanted to be around other people. As a doctor, the author examined how medicine was intent on prolonging life, with sometimes devastating consequences, when the body was ready to die.

What I gained most from Dr. Gawande's book was that I was in charge of my own healthcare. Doctors may recommend a pacemaker, but it was a recommendation. Doctors may prescribe antibiotics, but it was my choice to take them or not. If I was eighty years old and diagnosed with cancer, chemotherapy was up to me.

Doctors will do all they can to be proactive. We must have the final say—we must make our own decisions.

We also read *Dead Wake: The Last Crossing of the Lusitania* by Erik Larson. The history was very interesting, but I was struck by the interviews conducted with passengers who were pulled out of the North Atlantic and survived. Many said they would never fear death again. They experienced great peace in the frigid waters. I did not expect that.

In our culture, death is seen as a failure. I learned this from Joan Didion's book, *The Year of Magical Thinking*, about the year of numbness after she lost her husband. She said, "I realize how open we are to the persistent message that we can avert death. And its punitive correlative, the message that if death catches us we have only ourselves to blame."

It's true, isn't it? We offer "rah-rah" cheerleader phrases to the dying, urging them on, saying, "You can beat this!" If they didn't "beat" their illness, it could seem like a failure. Oh, if only they would have tried harder, or done this or that. Death was not the opposing NFL team.

I remember when my father had inoperable kidney cancer. During his last hospital stay, he said he didn't want extreme measures to keep him alive, and we were willing to respect his wishes. But when the doctor ordered a transfusion because my father was bleeding internally, we all agreed. Then Dad said, "Wait a minute. That is just what I do *not* want." He called the doctor and told him no transfusion. He died within a few days. That was taking charge of his own healthcare, and I admired the courage he showed.

When my mother had dementia, her quality of life completely diminished from the vital woman she had been, an artist and a writer, as well as a world traveler. She would have hated her final eighteen months. I asked my doctor how I should deal with "end of life" issues, and the advice he gave me was so helpful I hope to remember it for my own final days.

He said, "Pneumonia and sepsis (the result of the body's response to infection) are the body's ways of dying. They are normal. Do not treat pneumonia or sepsis when a person is at the end of their life."

And so, when mother received a diagnosis of sepsis later that year (probably originating from a urinary tract infection), I told the nursing home physician we would take no further measures. Amanda and I sat with her as she lay with her eyes closed, unable to speak. We told her she was one of the lucky ones who would get to die in her own bed with no tubes attached. We told her we would be with her until the end, and her headstone would say, "You Are My Sunshine." I almost felt her breathing lighten.

I still remember a doctor running up to me in the hallway at the nursing home and saying, "We isolated the bacteria. We can give her massive doses of antibiotics intravenously to fight the sepsis."

I shook my head no and looked at the floor. It was difficult to say no to medical professionals, especially when you couldn't be sure if you were doing the right thing.

Then, and only then, did he reach out and place a hand on my shoulder.

"You are doing the right thing," he said. "This is no quality of life for her."

I felt relieved, but also angry that he might have swayed me from letting nature take its course—all in the name of proactive medicine.

One of our former presidents was back in the hospital with pneumonia. He was over ninety years of age. Was it because of his importance as a former president that he was not allowed to die? Every effort was being made to keep him alive. I don't know if it was true or not, but someone told me former president Harry Truman suffered greatly in his final days because the medical establishment pulled out all of the technical stops to keep him alive—respirator, catheter, feeding tube, etc.

I don't know anyone who wants to die that way.

My minister at the Methodist church once said there was a correlation between living well and dying well.

"If you can trust others, you can trust God. If you have learned to forgive, you can believe you are forgiven. If you have learned to love, you can die in the certainty you are loved."

I have faith in the afterlife promised to us by Jesus, who said, "I go to prepare a room for you." Sometimes, we have to let go and trust. Knowing when that time was—that was the hard part.

***

It was not easy to admit I had an "after death" experience of seeing someone I loved, or to whom I was close, after they died. I knew it sounded a bit flaky. The deceased individual had many other friends and family who would have liked to experience closeness just once more. Why was I the one lucky enough to sense their presence? Others would have loved the reassurance of feeling their loved one's well being, and yet they had no such blessing.

I believe that very deep grief may prevent such experiences. The body and mind felt numb after death, and there was often shock. It might take weeks or months to begin to regain a sense of normalcy, or to finally let the grief set in.

In any case, I felt the presence of two individuals after their deaths, and, in both cases, it was on the day after they died. Both visits were brief, under thirty seconds in earth time. There have been other deaths when I did not experience any presence. For example, when my father died, I had no after-death experience from him. The same with my good friend, Gail.

My first experience occurred after my mother, Adrienne, died. Let me give some background first. As I mentioned, my family doctor told me that sepsis and/ or pneumonia were natural ways for the body to die and recommended not treating them for someone with dementia, like my mother.

When my mother developed sepsis, after conferring

with my three sisters and two uncles, I informed the staff we would take no further measures. Without food or IVs, death would come within three days, they said. The staff assured me that my mother would not feel thirst.

It was a massive burden to be responsible for the end of someone's life. Amanda was nineteen, and she and I stayed with her grandmother around the clock for three days. We sang hymns to her. She would not be alone, I told her, as I held her hand. Her funeral would be in Mississippi, as she wanted, and she would be buried near beloved relatives.

On the third day, her breathing became horrible and loud and she died. I had never been with a person while they were actively dying, and it wasn't what I expected. I expected her to sigh and die quietly. She would look like the same person, only asleep. Instead, as we held her hands, her body struggled through a noisy breath, and I was amazed to see a vortex of air spiraling around her mouth, which to me was when her soul left her body. After that, there was another horrible rattling breath, and her entire face was transformed.

As I watched in horror, I saw that, when her spirit

left, her body lost the life force of animation, and was changed as though a hand waved across her face. What was left bore no resemblance to my beautiful mother, but was more like Edvard Munch's rendition of *The Scream*. At that moment, I realized how ill her body had been. What was left was nothing like the mother I loved.

It seemed her spirit paused briefly up in the left-hand corner of the room and looked down on us. But that was brief, and her spirit seemed to be gone as I continued to look at what was left of the woman I had known and loved.

Someone called the funeral home—I can't remember who made the call. I had selected this particular business in advance because it was run by women, and soon two women arrived to pick up the body. I remember thinking the body bag they brought was quite lovely, and it looked like brown velvet. They kindly asked us if we wanted more time to sit with the body. I was a bit abrupt as I emphatically stated, "No!" feeling that the husk remaining on that bed bore no resemblance to my mother.

In grief, Amanda and I went home on that bleak November evening, a week before Thanksgiving. That night, she and I huddled together in my bed on the first floor. The upstairs rattled and creaked as high winds moaned around the house. We felt like Adrienne was shaking the rafters, and I wondered if she was angry about her death. It was a sleepless night.

The next morning, the winds calmed and the sun was out. I had an appointment at the funeral home to make the final arrangements. *My* spirit was very down, as the night had been full of terrors, and the death I witnessed was not beautiful, but ugly. Alone, I drove to the funeral home and parked. Although I chose this funeral home, I had never been to the business site.

As I walked along the sidewalk, an unexpected thing happened— I felt a younger version of my mother fall into step beside me. She was in her prime, probably as she had been in her twenties, and she walked with a vigorous and youthful step. I was in my fifties and walked with a bit of a hunch, but she skipped right along, just behind my shoulder. She seemed to be wearing an A-line skirt and flat shoes. I kept walking and did not look to the side to see her face because I was afraid she would leave.

We came up to the building which was a bit unusual

for Wisconsin: a white stucco, Spanish architecture style. This was very serendipitous because my mother loved southwestern architecture. We walked together up the stairs with the black wrought-iron railings, through the arched entry and the heavy oak door, and stepped into a spacious receiving area with bright, red, wool area rugs and dark wood beams. Beside me, I felt my mother say, "Oh! This is wonderful!" and then she left.

This "visit" from my mother obliterated the image of her death from my mind. The experience of her as vigorous, happy, and joyful was the greatest gift possible. I will always be grateful. It gave me a vision of what I think our lives will be like—we will be recognizable as the unique individuals we were, and the spiritual body will be whole, well, and vibrant.

My second experience was just as unexpected. For twenty years, Arthur and I were part of a fellowship group at our church. After our divorce, he moved to Illinois, but I continued to participate. Gary was quite a live wire in the group, always making everyone laugh. He was a "close talker" who often leaned in to tell a punch line or make a side joke in your ear.

Our group gathered for a potluck one Saturday, and I remember Gary helped me carry my glass 9x13 pans out to my Honda Civic before he jumped into his car and drove off.

When I received a phone call a few days later that he had died of a heart attack, it was a shock. I remember sitting in my cubicle at work the next day. I was having a hard time getting any work done. The computer program came up, but I still sat in my chair, doing nothing. In my head, I had a conversation with Gary, and I was chiding him. *What's the matter with you? Don't you know people have heart attacks all of the time and they just go to rehab for a while or have a stent put in, and then they're fine? How could you just die when you had no symptoms?*

Suddenly, I felt a light touch on my shoulder as Gary leaned in closer to tell me something.

"You won't believe how wonderful it is here," his voice murmured.

Then, he was gone. I sat there a moment longer, but then thought, *Well, that's that,* and I got back to work on my computer.

By the way, I mentioned I did not have any visits

from my father after he died. But my sister Pam had an odd experience. The week after he died, she received a teletype (remember those?) from a coworker/friend in another office. The message said, "Happy Valentine's Day, Pam. Love, Daddy."

My sister called her friend Maggie and asked her about the teletype.

"How did you sign it?" she asked.

"I just signed it 'Maggie,' why?" Maggie wondered.

"Well, it's signed 'Daddy,'" Pam explained.

Who knows what happened to that teletype message as it traveled through the air between offices. Weird.

Those were my two experiences. I hope they will help you feel less afraid of dying. They have certainly helped me.

Chapter 15
Mishaps and Melodies

Well, back to the business of living.

I used to know how to cook. Recently, procedures that were second nature have not turned out well—in fact, they have been disastrous.

For example, I wanted to make corn muffins. I had a brand new Teflon muffin pan. Scrounging through my cupboards, I could not find any cupcake liners. *Oh, well,* I thought, *it's a brand new Teflon pan, so it's non-stick.*

Wrong. I could have sprayed the pan with non-stick spray but didn't think I needed to. That's what I mean about how I used to know how to cook. In the days when I baked on a regular basis, I would not have made a mistake like that.

As you can guess, the corn muffins stuck to their little individual cups. I couldn't use a metal spoon to dig them out because I did not want to scratch my new pan, so I found a plastic knife from Wendy's and used that to pry them out. Even with my best efforts, I only got the top

157

half of each muffin. The bottom half got washed into the sink in a soggy, gritty, corn muffin mess. Next time I will remember the non-stick spray—I hope.

For Thanksgiving, I always make butterhorn crescent rolls. This year, the yeast proofed beautifully and the dough mixed together well. It sat in the refrigerator overnight and rose perfectly, so it looked like a great batch of butterhorns. I rolled the dough, basted it with melted butter, cut the triangles, and rolled them all up into crescent shapes. They even fit onto my four new Teflon baking sheets (which I sprayed with non-stick spray). Everything was going well.

The rolls needed to rise in a warm spot for an hour. Since I lived in a new apartment, I couldn't think of a warm spot that would be suitable. I once heard of heating the oven to 150 degrees for a few minutes, turning off the oven, and letting the dough rise in the oven. I thought I would try this. Usually, I covered the rolls with damp tea towels, but it was too bulky to put four pans in the oven that way. Instead, I dampened paper towels and placed them across each pan. The four pans fit in the oven, and I set the timer for one hour. After only forty minutes, the aroma of yeast was so strong I decided to check on them.

Pulling one pan out of the oven, I could see the rolls had already doubled in size. I tried to lift the paper towel off of this batch and found the dough was so soft and sticky, the paper had adhered to the rolls. I grabbed my kitchen scissors and cut away at the bits of dough as I lifted the paper towel. Then, I looked at the rolls. Instead of looking like my usual butterhorns, they looked like the giant soft white larva of some monstrous moth. Hideous.

Quickly, I pulled the other pans out and repeated the process, lifting stuck paper toweling off of the gooey, sticky rolls and cutting the globs away from the paper with my scissors.

Oh, well. Maybe the rolls would recover in the baking process.

I put all four pans into a 350 degree oven and baked them for fifteen minutes. You know what happened. The lower two pans charred on the bottom of the rolls. The two pans in the upper part of the oven weren't too bad, although their odd time rising in the oven, plus the stuck paper toweling, left them looking distorted and spiky.

What was I thinking? I used to know the lower pans

would burn on the bottom. How could I forget?

I made myself two sticky note reminders and put them on my recipe. "Do not put the rolls in the oven to rise," and "Only bake two pans at a time." There was a time when I would have known this, but next year I think I will need the sticky note reminders.

By the way, have you noticed that chili powder and cinnamon come in very similar looking bottles? But that's another story.

***

Whenever I ordered a special cake from the bakery, there was always that moment of anxiety when I went to pick it up—*Will it be ready? I hope they didn't lose my order.*

Bakers must take a course called, "How to Give Your Customer a Heart Attack." That day, the baker looked for my order among the cakes lined up on the baker's rack, stepped back into the oven area—nope, not there— started looking under dish towels and pot holders, and all while I held my breath.

Then, the lady in charge looked on the baker's rack again and found it.

"Wow, I must be blind," said the first gal.

With care, she placed the quarter-sheet cake in front of me, attractively boxed. After simultaneously scaring you that the cake wasn't ready and scarring you for life, they must hope you will take the cake, pay for it quickly, and leave. However, I looked through the clear plastic window to admire the decorations.

The cake was to honor a member of our writers' group who had been published fifty times over the past twenty years. That was quite an accomplishment, so when I phoned in the cake order I requested chocolate cake and chocolate frosting, which Shirley loved, to be decorated with balloons and the phrase, "20 Years of Writing!"

But when I gazed at the chocolate cake with red and yellow balloons, I noticed that in blue lettering, slanted across the cake, was the phrase:

"20 Years of Writting!"

I laughed out loud at the irony.

"Excuse me," I said, "But I am taking this to a *writers' group* and I cannot take it with a misspelled word."

The two ladies in the bakery looked at the cake in confusion. "What is the problem?" they asked.

I pointed out that "writing" should not have two T's. They frowned at me like I did not know what I was talking about.

"Trust me," I said. "'Writing' has one T."

"All we did is follow the written order." They showed me the paper with the order I phoned in. Yep. The paper showed 'writing' with two T's.

"I did not know I had to spell 'writing' when I phoned in the order," I explained.

Obviously, it was my fault.

We decided they could carefully lift off one blue frosting "t" and reconnect the 'i' and remaining 't' with a slightly wi-i-i-i-der bit of cursive. That worked pretty well.

They also gave me five dollars off of the cake. At the checkout, the clerk and I had a good laugh. She said, "Doesn't 'writing' have two T's?"

Mind you, these were not young kids, but older women I would have expected to know better.

I snapped a photo of the cake with the misspelling and

my writers' group loved the story. We aren't all natural spellers. We depend on spell check. But most importantly, the cake was delicious, and Shirley loved the chocolate frosting.

***

When you move to a new place, you try a variety of different things. Some you really like and decide to stick with them, and others are fine for a time but not something you choose to continue. Water exercise was still enjoyable. I had increased my time in the YMCA pool from two days a week to three, and I wanted to add a fourth. Some of the ladies went five days a week, but I couldn't see myself doing that.

Joanna was going to rehab for some knee problems. Her therapist told her, "Motion is lotion." I kept thinking of that as I "jogged" and "cross country skiied" in the water.

It really helped to have music accompany our exercise. I laughed that I was "rocking out" to "Runaround Sue" by Dion and the Belmonts. Or *"It's a darn good life when you've got a wife, like Honeycomb."*

I couldn't believe I still knew almost every word to that song, just as I did when it was popular over fifty years ago. Sixteen-year-old Nancy would not recognize me, but I remember her very well.

There I was, wearing a belt to keep me afloat and splashing along to the same music I loved as a teenager.

Back then, the gym was decorated with mermaids for the "Enchantment Under the Sea" themed Junior-Senior prom. In my older years, I really "fluttered" like a mermaid in the turquoise water of the YMCA pool. My school friends Dian, Barb, Ruth, and Liz had become Faye, Pat, Gladys, and Mabel.

But the Everly Brothers still made my heart sing.

In fact, the YMCA had become a great resource for exercise and community.

Our local Y has an Active Older Adults Director, Becky. She states, "Studies of aging adults show the direct relationship between good health and social connection, so in order to help adults age well, we have become intentional in our programming. The Y has always done a good job addressing the physical aspect of adult health, but we have expanded our programming to include the

Spirit & Mind components of the original Y vision of Spirit, Mind, & Body.

"For example, once a month we offer a lunchtime learning opportunity where members and non-members can gather together over lunch and interact, then listen to a speaker who presents about various topics of interest. Some of the topics we have addressed are: Brain Health, Photography, How to Choose a Kayak, and Understanding Nutrition Labels.

"Another aspect of our programming involves trips. Trying to reach all interests and levels of economic status, we offer opportunities to do things locally for very little money as well as those that will take us to Green Bay, the Twin Cities, Madison, and even overnight. These types of activities are incredibly important because this population went from interacting daily with other adults due to work or raising a family to not having an automatic means of communal participation. Our programming is trying to address this need and will continue to expand in all three areas (Spirit, Mind & Body) in order to help adults in our area to age well."

I was glad we had an active YMCA and so many

opportunities. Be sure to check out the programs in your area.

In addition to the Y, I was working with the Hmong children and enjoying them. Some had Hmong names and some had English names. I quizzed Philip on math facts. The third-grade girls let me ask them their spelling words. There seemed to be quite a few variations of a similar name: Angelina, Angel, Angela.

Andrew read to me from the library book, "What's Under Your Feet," about animals that burrowed in the ground. We talked about snakes "slithering" and chipmunks "scurrying." I learned something, too. I didn't know a prairie dog was called a 'dog' because of its barking call, even though it was a member of the squirrel family. Andrew bounced up and down as he read, and I thought it must be hard to go to homework club after a full day of school.

If I were to get on my soapbox, I would certainly advocate for children to get *more* exercise time at school, not less. When I was taking classes to learn about the insurance industry for work, the trainer said adult learners need a break every hour. And she was sure to provide a regular stretch break, snack time, or bathroom recess. Children need the same opportunities. Exercise clears the cobwebs and enables us to focus more.

Anyway, I might increase my time volunteering at this elementary school. The teachers could use the help.

One example of something I tried but gave up was singing in the church choir. I do love to sing. But the rehearsal time was 7:00-8:30 at night, which was after dark eight months of the year. Like many my age, I had given up driving after dark. So I made a joyful noise from the pew.

One of my neighbors asked me about my volunteer work. She said, "Well, I am not going to give my time for free. If someone wants to pay me, that's different."

This made me think of these words by Edward Everett Hale:

I am only one, but I am one.
I cannot do everything, but I can do something.
And I will not let what I cannot do interfere with what I
can do.

Chapter 16
So Long, Oolong

A few people asked me, "Nancy, what *don't* you like about your new living space?"

It was true; I tried to think positively. One of my life philosophies came from the Stoic, Epictetus. He said, "Every pitcher has two handles by which it can be borne." Think of a woman carrying a two-handled pitcher of water on her head. He meant that every circumstance can be considered from two points of view. It's up to us to choose which handle we grasp—the positive or the negative.

That said, I could still come up with a few things that had been an adjustment.

When I moved to Bentwood, I thought everyone would be like me, adjusting to a new community. I should have realized that many of the residents were from this area and already knew each other before they moved in. I did not expect that. It meant some residents already had built-in friendships. But not always. Those residents who had known each other for years may not have wanted to have much to do with each other anymore. It went both ways.

I did miss my bird feeders, though. But I remembered my accident in the snow when I went to refill them. And I understood the seeds were messy and attracted rodents.

My neighbor above me, Sheila, accidentally left her sink running. It overflowed and ran down my bathroom light, causing the fixture to crash onto the floor. Some of the water also ran down the wall between the dining room and bathroom. She felt so bad! The management here was very responsive and they repaired the damage promptly after the wall dried out. Everything was back to normal in about two weeks.

For the most part, though, I hardly knew my neighbors were there. The apartments were well insulated. (I saw the insulation when the ceiling collapsed . . . ha, ha.)

It would not have been my first choice to have carpet in the apartment. I had asthma, and carpeting held dust. In fact, I was concerned about being able to clean the carpet under my bed, so I came up with a good solution—I didn't have a bed. Yep, I put my box spring and mattress directly on the carpet, and I loved it. Mattresses are quite deep, so it didn't look strange when the quilt and pillows were on it. The "bed" was the perfect height for me when I sat down to put on my socks. And I didn't have to worry about cleaning under it.

Another disadvantage to living here—an ambulance arrived at least once a week. That was a natural consequence of living with a concentrated number of senior citizens. But when it happened in the middle of the night, it could be disconcerting and disruptive. And my neighbors told me to expect one or two deaths a year, although I had not experienced that yet. My daughter asked me if it was depressing to live where people were at the end of their lives. So far, I had not found it depressing. I liked being with people my age who experienced some of the same limitations I did.

I think everyone would agree the absolute worst thing about living here was the fire alarm test that occured every Wednesday morning at 10:00 in the morning. That alarm was so shrill I jumped right out of my socks. I tried to be out on Wednesday mornings, even though the alarm was only tested for a few seconds.

One time, lightning struck the building in a

thunderstorm and the alarm sounded non-stop for forty minutes. Two fire trucks and two ambulances responded. They needed to ascertain if there was a fire in the alarm panel and ensure the residents were safe before the alarm could be silenced.

Meanwhile, some senior citizens living on the second and third floors walked down the stairs, (like the sign on the elevator tells them to do), in their pajamas and robes and congregated in the parking lot on a drizzly evening. They could have gone to the basement, but, just like kids, they wanted to watch the emergency responders.

First-floor residents like me stepped out onto their patios with umbrellas and called to each other.

"That strike was right above my apartment!" numerous voices said from opposite ends of the building.

"I thought it was going to come right into the room."

"I hope the fire department gets here soon."

"Do you feel safe where you are? Come on over if you want company."

There was comfort in community during an emergency.

At last, blissful silence returned. No fire was found. The staff invited the residents for root beer floats the next day to celebrate the safe ending of a scary night.

Then the bad news: A new alarm system needed to be installed. We had to be ready for it to be tested at 3:00.

***

Mildred and Trudy were going to Florida and then on a cruise to the Bahamas. At coffee hour, Trudy told us about her preparations.

She withdrew six hundred dollars in cash for the trip and had the money in her purse in her apartment. When she was getting ready to come to coffee hour, Trudy felt anxious about leaving that much money just sitting there because she never locked her apartment. So she came up with a great idea: "I hid my purse way back in the linen closet. And I placed an empty decoy purse on the dining room table, so in case anyone opens my apartment door, they will grab the decoy." Well, we laughed at her ingenuity—even though it was unlikely someone would open her apartment door, let alone take anything. There had never been any theft in any of the apartments.

I got an update from Joanna. After coffee hour, when

Trudy returned to her apartment, the decoy purse was right where she left it. But the real purse with six-hundred dollars in it was not in the linen closet. She pulled all of the towels and sheets out but could not find it. Trudy called Mildred in a panic. Mildred went over and said, "You must have put it somewhere else." Of course, they argued for a while. Then Mildred looked in a different closet and found the purse there. Trudy could breathe again.

***

I've always been a frugal person. For example, I often bought groceries at a store where you bring your own bags and pack your own groceries. Why buy baby carrots when it was cheaper to buy a pound of carrots and cut them up? It must have been my Scottish ancestry that made me a penny pincher in most situations.

However, I once treated myself to Oolong tea from a specialty tea store. "Specialty" meant expensive. Legend has it that this tea was from leaves that grew so high that the Chinese monks trained monkeys to climb the tree and pick the leaves. I purchased a canister that was partially filled with the leaves, and I actually paid twenty-eight dollars for it! Yes, twenty-eight dollars for tea. I know it's hard to believe, but I enjoyed it immensely and savored every delicious drop. I still felt a little guilty, though, and couldn't say for sure that the tea was worth all that money.

Those leaves lasted me quite a while; but, when they were gone, I went back to more reasonably priced herbal blends and didn't think too much about it—until I was in a Milwaukee mall where I saw the exact same specialty tea shop that carried the Oolong tea.

Should I? Oh, why not.

So I went in and asked for the monkey-picked Oolong, and the associate lifted the tin container with reverence. On the side, I could see it was twenty-five dollars, and I thought, *That's about what I paid before.* She offered me a narrow canister or a larger size, and I said the narrow one would be fine. As she dipped the fragrant leaves into the airtight canister, we chatted about keeping the leaves fresh and how long to steep them.

The cash register was busy, so there was a delay while I waited to be checked out, and other customers lined up behind me. At last, she proceeded to ring me up and turned to me with a smile, announcing my purchase totaled one hundred and five dollars!

Well, I just about fainted. Immediately, the realization dawned. The tea cost twenty-five dollars *per ounce*! My previous purchase must have been for just *one ounce* of the monkey-picked leaves, and somehow I had a full canister of over four ounces.

One hundred and five dollars for *tea*! Who was I? Kim Kardashian?

Well, I was too embarrassed to admit my error, especially after waiting in line and with others queued behind me, so I paid for the leaves of gold with my credit card and smiled in what I hoped was a nonchalant manner. As I thought about my purchase for the rest of that day, I realized I should have said, "Oh, my. I had no idea it would be that expensive. I'll have to get a smaller amount."

That's called the school of hard knocks.

Every time I drank a cup of that tea, which was frequently (it *was* a full container, after all), I shook my head over my stupidity. The tea was good, but not *that* good. It's hard to enjoy something when you are experiencing "buyer's remorse." Good thing I chose the narrow canister rather than the fat one. Either way, Oolong tea made a monkey out of me.

***

Oh, we heard the most terrible news. Evangeline and Rupert died in an auto accident two days ago.

Their obituaries were in the newspaper—a full two columns. Of course, it *was* for both of them.

She and Rupert had four children. The obituary explained how their family cherished Evangeline and Rupert and what wonderful parents they were; perhaps one of the children wrote it.

Evangeline never met a craft she didn't like according to her obituary. She took ceramics to nursing home residents and helped them paint the green ware. She gifted hand-sewn quilts to her family. Her lemon meringue pie was famous.

I was surprised to read that Rupert had been a wonderful singer and sang in barbershop quartets most of his life. He was a frequent soloist in their Lutheran church, and sang "The Lord's Prayer" at his grandchildren's weddings. He loved to read and always carried a book with him.

Mr. and Mrs. were married more than sixty years. Their legacy included nine grandchildren and six great-grandchildren.

People forget that senior citizens had a life before they got old. We see them with dementia or a walker and that's all we see. The obituaries described a couple I would have liked to know better. I wish I had made more of an effort and been less impatient. Ah, still learning lessons at my late age.

Chapter 17
Happy Noon Year

I certainly felt fortunate that Amanda and I agreed on everything in life. Okay, that was intended as—well, not *sarcasm,* but definitely with an eye-roll.

A recent example—my daughter returned a gift to me that I gave her two years ago.

"Mom, thank you so much for these placemats, and they are lovely, but honestly they are just one more thing for me to wash."

You grandmothers out there might immediately understand why I gifted my daughter with placemats—because I could not understand how she fed her family dinner every night on a *bare table.* Perhaps I'm a little obsessive compulsive, but bare tables grated on my nerves.

So, two years ago when I found these especially nice placemats, I knew just who could use them, and I picked some up for my daughter-in-law Jane, too. They were a great memento from Maine, (how often had we read

Blueberries for Sal?), with blueberries printed on one side and a solid blue background on the other.

But my efforts were for naught. Oh, well, live and let live.

Over Christmas, my spirits lifted. I was talking with two other grandmothers about their holiday visit from the grandchildren. Both of them told me their children do not have a dinnertime meal with the family when they are in their own home. Everyone just sort of grazes when they are hungry, apparently. So naturally it was different when they ate at Grandma's, and everyone was expected to sit down at the same time.

Well, I felt quite superior. Both my daughter-in-law and daughter served regular family dinners—even if it was usually on a bare table. And, I have to admit, I really wanted those placemats for myself, anyway.

Being the parent of adult children means letting them live their own lives. Somewhere, I heard this saying: "You can never be fully yourself until after your parents are gone."

It doesn't have to be that way. I want my children free to be themselves now, before I am gone.

The words of Kahlil Gibran were a great help to me when my children were young:

Your children are not your children.
They are the sons and daughters of life's longing for itself.
They come through you, but not from you.
And though they are with you, yet they belong not to you.

You may house their bodies, but not souls.

You may strive to be like them, but seek not to make them like you.
You are the bows from which your children as living arrows are sent forth.

The Archer sees the mark upon the path of the infinite, and He bends you with His might
That his arrows may go swift and far.
Let your bending in the archer's hand be for gladness;
For even as He loves the arrow that flies, so He loves also the bow that is stable.

I loved the idea that they came through us, but did not

belong to us. They might look like us, but they were their own souls. And the line, "You may strive to be like them, but seek not to make them like you" was true; I have learned so much from my children and I did strive to be like them. I admired their humor, their warmth, their engagement with life. Parents could learn from their children. We were just the bows that sent them forth.

The last line really resonated with me:

"For even as He loves the arrow that flies, so He loves also the bow that is stable."

The Archer, who I take to be God, loved me as I bent in His hand, to send my children forth—without placemats.

***

Elaine used to type sermons for a Jehovah's Witness pastor. Ruth raised turtles in plastic shoe boxes. A part of Joanna's intestine was stored at the local university.

Those are interesting facts I learned about my neighbors at my Noon Year's Eve Party. That's a party to celebrate the New Year at noon. I heard about the idea from a friend in Minneapolis, and an online search revealed noon celebrations had become a new fad, especially at public libraries. Perfect for seniors who didn't want to be out at midnight.

It was a bit spur-of-the-moment, but I invited ten ladies from Bentwood and gave quite a bit of thought to where everyone would sit. Ten was certainly my apartment's maximum. Everyone replied that they could come.

Then I thought, *Better make room in my coat closet. It is January, after all. But, Oh! No need to clear out the closet. No one will be wearing coats since they can just walk over in the building.*

No coats, no boots—how wonderful!

Many of the ladies brought leftover Christmas goodies, so my original simple refreshments became quite a spread—smoked turkey and rolls, baguettes, crackers and dip, shrimp, veggie trays, chicken salad, and assorted chocolates.

After we ate, we played *Taboo*, and it was just-for-fun with no teams and no winners or losers. *Taboo* was a fun parlor game, similar to charades, only with talking. You tried to get the group to guess the word on the card you chose, but certain clues were "taboo." For example, you might draw a card with the word "house." That seemed simple enough, but the additional directions stated you could not use the word "live," "residence," or "abode," as you tried to get the group to guess your word. Elaine was very clever. She said, "A chicken coop is a hen's _____." Someone guessed "house" and then it was their turn to draw a card.

Everyone got into the festive spirit. After we each had two turns, Roberta suggested we play *Two Truths and a Lie*. In that game, you told two things about yourself that were true and then you totally made up the last one; but of course, you tried to tell two things that were really odd that were true, just to throw people off. Then people had to guess which one was the lie.

That's how I found out Elaine used to type the Jehovah's Witness sermons. That seemed like a "lie," since it was so strange, but it was true. Elaine used to be a secretary, and you know how "back in the day" the bosses asked secretaries to take on extra duties that were not in their job description? Elaine's boss was also a minister in the Jehovah's Witness church, and he asked her to type his sermons. She couldn't say 'no,' of course.

In addition, Roberta raised turtles in the elementary school classroom where she taught fifty first graders at a parochial school, and Joanna had emergency surgery when she was two. Believe it or not, she swallowed an open safety pin and lived to tell the tale. She also tried to tell her grandmother, as best as a two-year-old could talk, what she did, and her grandmother finally understood. That was when cloth diapers were fastened with safety pins, and little Joanna undid a pin when she was supposed to be napping. You know children that age put everything in their mouths. Children's Hospital was associated with the university at that time, and a section of Joanna's intestine was still preserved in some lab there—maybe with a safety pin in it.

Now, these were not the normal, everyday things you learned about someone when you said, "I'm glad to meet you." We all enjoyed discovering interesting tidbits about each other's lives.

These ten women were all new friends from the apartment community—some in book group, some bridge players, and some neighbors from my floor. We raised a toast at noon and wished we might all gather again next year.

The year is behind me. So much has changed since I moved here—to a new town and new home. The best thing is—I am no longer alone. We early birds are happiest when we flock together.

Resources

For continued learning:

The Great Courses -

http://www.thegreatcourses.com

Call 800-832-2412 to request a catalog

Big Think -

https://www.youtube.com/user/bigthink

Free YouTube videos on interesting subjects

Yale University free courses -

http://oyc.yale.edu/

All lectures were recorded in the Yale College classroom and are available in video, audio, and text transcript formats. Registration is not required.

EDX -
https://www.edx.org/course?availability=Self-Paced
Various universities offer many free courses for online learning—You can choose "self-paced" and then a variety of subjects such as "art and culture," "history," "literature," and much more.

For general help with aging issues:

National Association of Senior Move Managers -
https://www.nasmm.org/
877-606-2766
For help downsizing.

Transitions with Jean-Jean Long Monteufel -
www.transitionswithjean.com
920-734-3260
Help with dealing with "all the stuff." It may be "stuff" in the home or emotional issues that come with downsizing. "You are not alone."

National Association of Area Agencies on Aging - https://www.n4a.org/
Enter your ZIP code to receive a listing of agencies near you.

For legal assistance:

AVVO Lawyer Directory - https://www.avvo.com/elder-law-lawyer.html
Find Law - http://lawyers.findlaw.com/lawyer/practice/elder-law
To locate an attorney specializing in elder law.

For information on long-term care insurance:

American Association for Long-Term Care Insurance - http://www.aaltci.org/
818-597-3227

Acknowledgements

Thank you to Mary Kautz, Nancy Jesse, and Patty A. O'Hara for reading my original manuscript and making suggestions. I am grateful to Jill Swenson of Swenson Book Development for her coaching and help developing my book proposal. My editor at Orange Hat Publishing, Christine Woods, helped me stay focused on the purpose for my book and is a verb-tense guru. Bruce Cochran, the talented cover artist from Prairie Village, KS, also happens to be my beloved uncle. And many thanks to all my friends at "Bentwood Hills," who know who they are.

About the Author

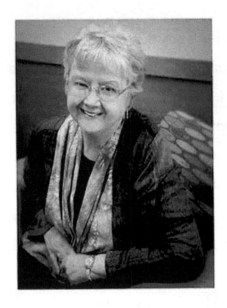

Nancy Runner lives and writes in Wisconsin, her home for the past 40 years. Her family includes two grown children, their spouses, and four grandchildren. Long ago, Nancy graduated from Coe College in Cedar Rapids, Iowa. In her growing up years, she lived in five states as well as England and Argentina. On nosy application forms, she checks the boxes for married, single, and divorced. Over her lifetime, she has learned change provides opportunity.

In her essays, Nancy explores relationships and their long term consequences, good and bad. Personal mishaps find their way into her writing: from getting stuck in the gas station car wash, to accidentally drinking the water from a vase of flowers, or paying over one hundred dollars for a canister of tea, Nancy likes to laugh at herself and hopefully provide encouragement to others.

Her books include, *2Cute 2Be 4Gotten*, *A Book about Mourning Doves*, *From Castles and Bombs to Nazis and Frauleins,* and *Early Birds Flock Together.*

www.nancyrunner.com

CPSIA information can be obtained
at www.ICGtesting.com
Printed in the USA
FFHW02n0117250818
47952436-51652FF